HOMEOPATHY
for
MUSCULOSKELETAL
HEALING

To Mary & John

Maybe, just maybe
this will help a little.

Merry Christmas

Marcia

HOMEOPATHY
for
MUSCULOSKELETAL
HEALING

Asa Hershoff N.D., D.C.

North Atlantic Books
Berkeley, California

Homeopathic Educational Services
Berkeley, California

Homeopathy for Musculoskeletal Healing

Published by
North Atlantic Books   Homeopathic Educational Services
P.O. Box 12327   2036 Blake St.
Berkeley, CA 94712   Berkeley, CA 94704

Figure photograph by David A. Wagner, courtesy of Merck & Co., Inc.
Cover illustration by Asa Hershoff
Cover design by Asa Hershoff and Legacy Media, Inc.
Book design and illustrations by Asa Hershoff
Printed in the United States of America

Homeopathy for Musculoskeletal Healing is sponsored by the Society for the Study of Native Arts and Sciences, a nonprofit educational corporation whose goals are to develop an educational and crosscultural perspective linking various scientific, social, and artistic fields; to nurture a holistic view of the arts, sciences, humanities, and healing; and to publish and distribute literature on the relationship of mind, body, and nature.

Library of Congress Cataloging-in-Publication Data
Hershoff, Asa, 1948–
    Homeopathy for musculoskeletal healing / Asa Hershoff.
       p. cm.
    Includes index.
    ISBN 1-55643-237-2
    1. Musculoskeletal system—Diseases—Homeopathic treatment.
  I. Title.
    RX261.R4H47   1996
    616.7'06—dc20   96-38435
                                                      CIP

1 2 3 4 5 6 7 8 9 / 99 98 97 96

To Doctor John Laplante, an extraordinary
healer who taught me about homeopathy
and about living in awareness.

CONTENTS

Condition Charts

Headache

MATERIA MEDICA

THERAPEUTIC GUIDE

APPENDIX

RESOURCES 299

BIBLIOGRAPHY 301

INDEX

Introduction

The Purpose of this Book

Musculoskeletal problems are the most pervasive and debilitating conditions in our culture, causing untold pain, disability, and just downright inconvenience. Possibly because low back pain, migraine, or a sore neck are not life-threatening, we tend to think that they are just a fact of life for which we expect no cure, and only little relief. Though medical drugs offer temporary alleviation of most musculoskeletal symptoms, both the underlying causes and potential cure of these conditions remains elusive. Homeopathy can contribute much to this situation, offering real and lasting cure using safe, natural, and effective remedies.

Homeopathy has long concerned itself with the practical business of getting sick people well, based on careful observation and scientific investigation of the healing process. Its philosophy and practice form a unified whole, a cohesive system that has demonstrated its effectiveness for two centuries, without need for major revision. Though homeopathic knowledge keeps expanding incrementally, it is not at the expense of previous information. It is a consistent and congruent system of care. Why? Because from its inception it was based on biological facts, on how the body and mind really express illness, how the organism attempts to heal itself, and how this process can be assisted.

Homeopathy has a remarkable record for treating and curing musculoskeletal conditions. This vital information is scattered throughout the vast treasury of homeopathic literature and clinical experience of 200 years. Though this body of knowledge is profound in its range and depth, books focusing on musculoskeletal treatment have been rare, and what does exist is dated or inadequate in various ways.

The present book is an attempt to gather and consolidate this wealth of knowledge and practical guidance and to present it in a highly accessible form. Each remedy discussed was researched in more than 150 books. This proved to be somewhat like wading into an equatorial jungle trying to carve out a clear and definite path through this maze of minute detail, and subtle differences in opinion. Ideally, the result balances a concise format with accurate and complete information. The traditional style of describing remedies is updated with modern terminology and physiology wherever possible, without losing the person-centered (rather than disease-centered) approach of homeopathy. For contemporary seekers of a natural, non-invasive, and human-scale medicine, the effects of simple, non-toxic homeopathic remedies can be easily verified.

HOW TO USE THIS BOOK

The layout of this book is influenced by my interest in graphic arts, multimedia, and the way people scan and assimilate knowledge in this information age. Designed as a rapid guide to finding the effective homeopathic remedies for a wide range of musculoskeletal conditions, this book provides accurate information with an easy-to-use interface. The book consists of four main sections and an appendix to offer a practical method of finding the correct curative remedy for various conditions. Each section has a standardized format as explained below.

1. PRINCIPLES OF HOMEOPATHY

In 16 main Topics or Chapters, this overview of homeopathic principles examines some of the key concepts necessary to intelligently prescribe a remedy. Not meant to be a complete course in homeopathy, it nevertheless provides a general understanding and a basis for further learning. Advanced practitioners may find interest in the way in which these principles are explained and visually illustrated.

2. CONDITION CHARTS

The thirty-one Condition Charts are related to specific musculoskeletal conditions or major areas of the body. A synopsis of the six to eight main remedies remedies for the condition or location are described and are linked numerically to more extensive descriptions in the Materia Medica. Some charts also provide illustrations of body areas and their associated homeopathic remedies..

3. MATERIA MEDICA

The Materia Medica contains descriptions of the sixty-one important musculoskeletal remedies found in the Condition Charts. The symptoms and modalities are a distillation of the essential characteristics of the remedies described in homeopathic literature. The main focus is the musculoskeletal symptoms of the remedy, with brief descriptions of their other characteristic symptoms of mind and body.

4. THERAPEUTIC GUIDE

This section provides more extensive lists of conditions and locations, and the remedies that can be effective for them, graded according to their relative importance.

5. APPENDIX

The relationship and interaction among the remedies described in this book are charted here, indicating the effective sequence for their use.

In HOMEOPATHY...

Successful prescribing is based on accurately matching the patient's unique symptoms to the medicines that will stimulate inherent physiological and biological healing mechanisms.

CONDITION CHARTS

To simplify the process, Condition Charts provide a comparison of the most useful remedies in the treatment of Low Back Pain, Headache, Arthritis, and other common conditions. For a more detailed analysis, each remedy in the flow chart is keyed to a full description of the medicine in the Materia Medica.

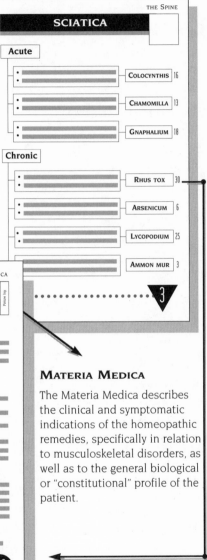

THE SPINE

SCIATICA

Acute

COLOCYNTHIS 16

CHAMOMILLA 13

GNAPHALIUM 18

Chronic

RHUS TOX 30

ARSENICUM 6

LYCOPODIUM 25

AMMON MUR 3

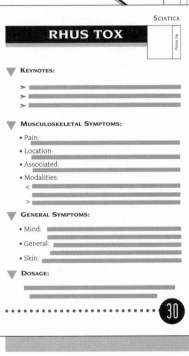

SCIATICA

RHUS TOX

▼ KEYNOTES:
>
>
>

▼ MUSCULOSKELETAL SYMPTOMS:
• Pain:
• Location:
• Associated:
• Modalities:
    <
    >

▼ GENERAL SYMPTOMS:
• Mind:
• General:
• Skin:

▼ DOSAGE:

30

MATERIA MEDICA

The Materia Medica describes the clinical and symptomatic indications of the homeopathic remedies, specifically in relation to musculoskeletal disorders, as well as to the general biological or "constitutional" profile of the patient.

ABOUT THE CONDITION CHARTS

CONDITION DESCRIPTION

The introductory page of each chart gives a brief discussion of the condition or location, describes the homeopathic approach to the problem, and suggests the psychological meaning of symptoms in this body area.

CONDITION CHARTS

These charts are designed to provide rapid access to the correct remedy for a variety of musculoskeletal conditions or anatomical locations. There can be dozens or even hundreds of remedies for some illnesses. Here we are focusing on the six to eight remedies that are most commonly found to be effective for that particular body area or condition. The standard features of the Condition Chart pages are outlined below and in the illustration opposite.

CONDITION TITLE

The charts are titled after commonly seen clinical syndromes such as Headache or Sciatica, or for a specific area, such as the Cervical Spine. In homeopathy one does not treat the diagnostic label, but the symptom-picture. Thus, the Low Back Pain Chart may be useful whether the underlying problem is disc disease, poor posture, or a recurrent strain.

SUBHEADINGS

Subheadings are used to further streamline the process of remedy selection, and the remedies may be arranged in a designated order.

PATIENT / REMEDY SYMPTOMS

The leading indications, keynotes, locations, and modalities (factors which improve or worsen the symptoms) of each remedy are described. These indications lead one to the name of the remedy that corresponds to the symptoms, and that can help cure the person who has them.

MATERIA MEDICA PAGE NUMBER

The number following each remedy is a reference to a detailed description of the medicine in the Materia Medica section. These are not page numbers, but the *remedy numbers*, prominently displayed on each page of the Materia Medica.

TYPICAL CONDITION CHART

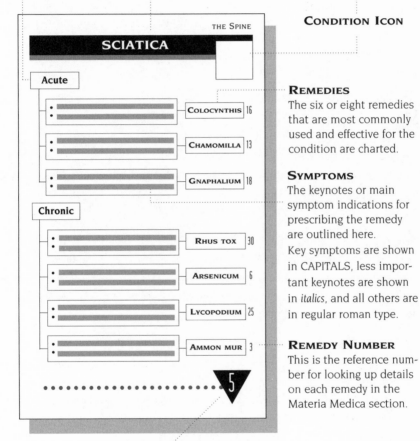

SUBHEADINGS
Wherever possible, the remedies are further categorized.

CONDITION
A specific condition or body area is the theme for each flow chart.

CONDITION ICON

REMEDIES
The six or eight remedies that are most commonly used and effective for the condition are charted.

SYMPTOMS
The keynotes or main symptom indications for prescribing the remedy are outlined here.
Key symptoms are shown in CAPITALS, less important keynotes are shown in *italics*, and all others are in regular roman type.

REMEDY NUMBER
This is the reference number for looking up details on each remedy in the Materia Medica section.

CHART NUMBER
Each chart has its own number, separate from the page number.

The Condition Chart section also has a number of diagrams that graphically illustrate the relationships and affinities of remedies to various conditions and areas of the body.

ABOUT THE MATERIA MEDICA

Homeopathic texts usually describe remedies in an extensive form, including symptoms of each organ system, and the broad variety of physical and emotional states. This approach is essential for comprehensive or "constitutional" prescribing — matching the entire person to his or her appropriate remedy. However, when prescribing for specific or local conditions, this may give us too much irrelevant information, and not enough data about the particular condition that is causing the pain and suffering. This book describes remedies in relation to the musculoskeletal system, and the conditions for which they are most effective, as related to the flow charts in the Condition Chart section.

MATERIA MEDICA

- Materia medica are the texts that describe the substances used in the practice of medicine, herbology, or homeopathy, etc. Homeopathic materia medica differ from the others in that they emphasize the detailed *symptoms of the patient*, rather than the physiological effects of a drug or its pathological indications.
- The key features of each homeopathic medicine or remedy are outlined in a systematic way, closely paralleling the way a homeopathic case history is taken in musculoskeletal conditions.
- To help the reader navigate through this information quickly and efficiently, this materia medica has a standardized two-page format. Details about the set-up of these pages are given below and demonstrated graphically in the accompanying diagrams.
- The REMEDY NAME used in the heading of the first page of each remedy is the one in common everyday use by homeopaths.
- The full LATIN NAME is used as the heading for the second page of each remedy description.
- A LINE DRAWING is included to give a more direct sense of the plant, animal, or mineral substance as a living, dynamic force, rather than a lifeless chemical ingredient or agent.
- The common ENGLISH NAMES are given next to each drawing.
- The Latin, English, and common name used by homeopaths are listed together for convenience at the front of the Materia Medica section.

KEYNOTES

The Keynotes section gives the essential indications of the remedy for rapid reference and easy recall.

SPECIFIC SYMPTOMS

Musculoskeletal symptoms are described under as many of the following headings as are applicable:

- PAIN: The quality and type of pain for which the remedy is most indicated, e.g. stitching, sore, bruised, sharp, etc. (see Condition Chart 1).
- LOCATION: Areas, locations, and tissues most affected by the remedy, the direction the pain may travel, areas of referred pain, etc.
- ASSOCIATED: Important symptoms or signs which may occur along with the pain or even be more prominent, including stiffness, joint deformity, heat or swelling, chilliness, etc. (see Condition Chart 2).
- ONSET: The time and / or conditions that initiate painful symptoms.
- CAUSE: Relevant causative factors such as injury, overexertion, etc.
- MODALITIES: Factors that make symptoms worse or better (indicated by the symbols < and > respectively), which may include:
— *Environment*: effects of heat, cold, weather changes, damp, open air.
— *Spatial*: effects of position, posture, motion, rest, specific activities.
— *Time*: specific time of day or night, cycle of recurrence, etc.
— *Sensory*: effects of sound, light, touch, pressure, and so on.
Modalities are explained in detail in Topic 6 in the Principles section.

SYMPTOM PROFILE

- The symptom profile helps to determine the "fit" of the remedy to the individual's metabolic and psychological type, e.g. their "constitution."
- Useful keynotes and leading symptoms are described for relevant organ systems and body locations using the following headings:
- PSYCHOLOGICAL SYMPTOMS: The intellectual and emotional profile is an important component of any remedy, including acute or chronic states or tendencies toward depression, anxiety, irritability, etc.
- METABOLIC SYMPTOMS: May include body morphology, disease tendencies, physical characteristics, temperature and climate sensitivities.
- ORGAN SYSTEMS: Other areas, symptoms or conditions strongly influenced by the remedy are briefly mentioned in order to give a more complete sense of the full range and characteristics of the medicine.
- DOSAGE: Typical potencies, frequency and suggested duration of administration are described. General guidelines and information on dose and potency are found in Topic 14 of the Principles section.

TYPICAL MATERIA MEDICA PAGES

Each remedy is described in a two-page format as follows:

REMEDY PICTURE

COMMON NAME
English name of the remedy.

REMEDY NAME
The name usually used by homeopaths.

KEYNOTES
The leading indications of the remedy for rapid reference.

MUSCULOSKELETAL SYMPTOMS
Symptoms relative to the musculoskeletal system are described according to type of pain and its onset, typical locations, causes, associated symptoms, and modalities.

Key symptoms are shown in CAPITALS, less important keynotes are shown in *italics*, and all others are in regular roman type.

MATERIA MEDICA

ARNICA

Mountain Daisy

▼ **KEYNOTES:**

➤
➤
➤

▼ **MUSCULOSKELETAL SYMPTOMS:**

Pain:

Location:

Causes:
Associated:

Modalities:
<
>

8

REMEDY NUMBER
Each remedy is numbered *separately from the page number*, and keyed to the Conditions Charts.

The second page of each remedy is designed as follows:

LATIN NAME
The full Latin name of the plant, mineral, or animal remedy.

General category of conditions treated by the remedy.

SYMPTOM PROFILE
The general and psychological profile of the homeopathic remedy (or patient requiring it), and a brief description of any relevant or important symptoms in areas other than the musculoskeletal system

DOSAGE
Suggestions for potency and repetition of the dose are briefly outlined.

CONDITIONS
The musculoskeletal conditions for which the remedy is commonly prescribed and effective are listed.

TRAUMA

ARNICA MONTANA

▼ SYMPTOM PROFILE

Psychological:

Metabolic:

Digestive:

Respiratory:

▼ DOSAGE:

Potency:

Repetition:

▼ CLINICAL CONDITIONS:

DIAGRAMS
Where applicable, and where space permits, additional diagrams help show the locations and symptoms of the remedy.

ABOUT THE THERAPEUTIC GUIDE

This section gives a complete listing of the remedy choices for various conditions, and also shows the therapeutic range of some of the important remedies. Generally the Guide is limited to the sixty-one remedies discussed in this book. Occasionally additional remedies are listed, if they are important remedies to consider for the problem.

ICON
An icon of a tissue or body area speeds the visual search.

LOCATION
The Guide is set up according to location, beginning with general tissues, then listing areas of the spine, and finally the extremities, from the upper limbs to the lower limbs, joint by joint.

CONDITIONS
The most common and typical conditions encountered in the area are listed alphabetically.

THERAPEUTIC GUIDE 285

BONE

BONE PAIN
Pulsatilla, RUTA, Calc carb, Calc phos, Chamomilla, Colocynthis, *Fluoric acid*, Lycopodium, MERCURIUS, Nat sulph, Phosphorus, Phytolacca, Sepia, Silicea, Staphysagria, Sulphur, Symphytum

BONE SPURS/OSTEOPHYTES/NODOSITIES
Causticum, Calc carb, Calc phos, CALC FLUOR, Caulophyllum, CAUSTICUM, *Colchicum*, Dulcamara, *Formica rufa*, Guaiacum, HECLA LAVA, *Phytolacca*, Rhododendron, RUTA, Rhus tox (for symptoms only; will not remove spurs), Silicea, Stellaria. (Lachnantes, Gnaphalium)

GROWING PAINS
Calc carb, CALC PHOS, Causticum, *Cimicifuga*, Colchicum, GUAIACUM, PHOSPHORIC ACIDUM, Phosphorus, Strontium carb, Silicea

REMEDIES
Remedies that are most effective for the condition are listed alphabetically. The standard notation for indicating the relative importance of the remedy is used:

All capitals indicates a remedy of the highest or 1st degree or grade.

Roman Italics indicates remedies of the 2nd degree.

Regular roman letters indicate remedies of the 3rd or least degree.

ARNICA, *Causticum*, Cimicifuga

However, the *right* remedy is the one that matches the symptom pattern, regardless of what grade it is!

Principles
of
Homeopathy

1. HOMEOPATHIC PRINCIPLES

HOMEOPATHIC MEDICINE

- Successful homeopathic treatment results in an overall increase in health and well-being, vitality, mental clarity, peace of mind, and a reaffirmation of one's personal creativity and freedom.
- Homeopathy recognizes the person as an integrated whole, and is designed to correct the disturbances that exist on physical, emotional, mental, and spiritual levels.
- The effects of homeopathic remedies and the way in which they are prescribed is radically different from that of mainstream medical drugs, and this is reflected in different understandings about the nature of health and illness.
- Homeopathy is based on a comprehensive set of principles and methods that ensures its effectiveness. These principles are not dry or abstract theories, but *practical* and *essential* roadmaps to using the remedies effectively.
- They are based on original discoveries, insights and observed facts about how the body and mind *actually heals itself*, and how the correct influences can release, augment, and accelerate these processes.
- The principles behind homeopathy have been tested, verified, and refined over two centuries by millions of homeopaths, their patients, and by people worldwide, using the remedies for simple home care.
- This first section will outline these principles and their practical application for successfully using homeopathic remedies.

SCOPE OF HOMEOPATHY

ACUTE CONDITIONS

- Acute conditions are defined by their depth and duration. They are of recent onset and abruptly, over a matter of hours or days. By definition, acute states are self-limited; if they last longer than a few days or a week, they are considered subacute or chronic. Homeopathy is extremely effective for acute swelling, pain, injury, inflammation, fevers, and other intense conditions, reducing the symptoms while promoting tissue repair and preventing long-term consequences or *sequelae*. In fact, homeopathy first achieved fame during the late 1800's during the acute and devastating epidemics of Europe and America, where it proved remarkably curative.

CHRONIC DISEASE

Generally "chronic" means lasting a long time, with no real resolution, and having a tendency to get slowly and progressively worse. Chronic conditions may arise after an acute illness that does not fully resolve itself, or they may arise insidiously over months or years. From a homeopathic point of view, chronic also means *deep-seated*, and arising from an underlying pattern of susceptibility or *miasm*. In homeopathy, these deep chronic patterns (miasms), whether genetic or acquired, are considered to be the underlying cause of progressive deterioration and of specific *styles* and *locations* of disease. While mainstream medicine provides only symptomatic relief or slowing of the process of chronic disease, homeopathy and other natural therapies have the possibility of repairing damaged tissues and curing chronic disease at a deeper level of the organism.

CONSTITUTIONAL PRESCRIBING

Constitutional homeopathy treats the person as a totality, in which symptoms of body and mind are perceived as a seamless whole. A remedy that benefits the core of the individual benefits all the parts. Classical homeopathy attempts to find the remedy that will match all aspects of the person: their metabolic and psychological make-up, their body type and genetic predispositions, their disease history, and their current symptom picture. Homeopathy is thus applicable whether disease symptoms are present or not. It is the ultimate *preventive medicine*, eradicating or neutralizing the patterns of susceptibility and tendency long before they express themselves as a specific illness.

LOCAL TREATMENT

Homeopathy is also capable of treating local problems or conditions. In cases of advanced degeneration, such as arthritic deformity in the hands or feet, it is necessary to work intensively on the local area. When an individual is strong, adaptive, and responsive, the whole organism can change through constitutional treatment. The more aged, devitalized, weakened, or damaged the organism is overall, the less likely it is to respond to deep constitutional change. Very gradual and local treatment becomes essential.

PALLIATION

- In advanced disease, such as cancer and intractable pain, and where cure may no longer be possible, homeopathy can often alleviate symptoms (palliation) and provide real physical and mental relief.
- Homeopathy can aid the dying, helping people navigate this time of spiritual transition with increased clarity, strength, and serenity.

COMPLEMENTARITY

Homeopathy can be used beneficially in conjunction with literally any mainstream or alternative therapy. However, it is the experience of homeopaths that some medical drugs can diminish or block the action of homeopathic medicines, while other drugs seem to have little influence on the effectiveness of remedies. Though drugs that strongly influence the nervous or immune system can be cited, it is a fairly individual situation, depending both on the person and their current medication. On the other hand, since homeopathic remedies work *with* the body to promote health and normal function, they do not interfere with stronger, relatively toxic medical drugs, which act forcefully or invasively. However, homeopathic remedies can diminish the side-effects of many drugs, i.e, homeopathic *Ipecac* decreases the nausea caused by certain cancer drugs or chemotherapy.

PHYSICAL

Homeopathy has an impact on the chemical, cellular, and structural health of the organism. Since it works with biological intelligence, it can reach the deepest, most subtle levels of anatomy and physiology.

EMOTIONAL

In general, homeopathy places great emphasis on our inner emotional life and its expression in feelings and relationships. Improvement in personal functioning and mental wellness is a touchstone and monitor of how effective a remedy is, even when treating physical ailments. While homeopathy works exceptionally well for acute states of grief, rage, or depression, it is also capable of helping change long-term patterns of emotional dysfunction, including issues of self-esteem, abuse, or loss of self. Recognized mental conditions such as bipolar disorders (manic depression), anxiety disorders, and ADHD, are prime candidates for homeopathic treatment, especially in conjunction with psychotherapy. During constitutional treatment old emotional memories may arise, unresolved issues can surface and be dealt with, and important changes in relationships, career, and life direction often occur.

TRANSPERSONAL

Homeopathy is a remarkable tool for spiritual growth and personal transformation, assisting in the long and sometimes arduous work on oneself that is required for self-development. The essence of homeopathic treatment is to free the person — mind and body — from fixed patterns. This includes limited patterns of perception and function, and the belief systems which shape experience. Remedies can reveal and set free long-hidden parts of ourselves.

2. HOMEOPATHY IN CONTEXT

We live in a unique time, with an immense range of natural healing methods and resources available to us. Some are new, while others are ancient (Ayurveda, acupuncture). In spite of widely different cultural roots, they share common themes that define them as natural, non-invasive, person-centered medicine. In this section we will explore some of the key concepts (such as the Principle of Similars and Infinitesimal Dose) that express homeopathy's unique place among these therapies.

THE SPECTRUM OF THERAPIES

Looking at the full spectrum of natural therapies, each one has a significant role to play in healing the body and mind. The example of building a house provides an analogy for the special capabilities and scope of each therapy, relative to homeopathy. *All of these therapies can influence the whole body.* The diagram on the next page indicates the "entry-point" or focus of the therapeutic method, its beginning point.

STRUCTURAL

- Biomechanical therapies, such as massage, chiropractic, and reflex therapies, work via the musculoskeletal, circulatory, and nervous structures in order to influence local and general health.
- There are many other body-centered systems that seek to alter emotional, energetic, and functional patterns through structural change.
- Structure is analogous to the *foundation* on which a house is built.

BIOCHEMICAL

- Biochemical therapy includes the broad science of nutrition and diet, including vitamin and mineral supplements, food concentrates, etc.
- These nutrients provide the *raw materials* on which all body functions and the life process itself depend, like the wood, nails, and cement of our house.

BIOLOGICAL

- Biological treatments stimulate organs, tissues, and cells to function optimally and to correct imbalances in physiology. They promote the natural process of detoxification and tissue regeneration.
- Biological therapies include herbal or botanical medicines and extracts, hydrotherapy, and various fasting or detoxifying methods.
- This is analogous to putting *workers* and their *tools* to work. Otherwise, even the finest building materials remain just a pile of separate objects.

ENERGETIC
- Homeopathy is a form of Energy Medicine, or "information medicine."
- According to the remedy strength or potency, homeopathy can work specifically on the material / biochemical level, or on increasingly subtler levels of information and biological intelligence.
- Acupuncture works directly with energy, moving it to or from areas of deficiency or excess. Many forms of psychic healing work similarly.

PATTERNS
- Continuing the analogy, raw materials, workers, tools, and adequate energy can create a lot of activity, but a house does not automatically come into existence.
- What is required, above all, is a blueprint, a plan that organizes all the elements into a meaningful and purposeful whole.
- Homeopathy excels at the level of pattern, software, or information technology — the level of biological intelligence. Though we can change the patterns of our behavior, lifestyle, or eating habits on a gross level, homeopathy can change the deepest patterns of biochemical, physiological, and even cellular function.
- Homeopathy frees the system from fixed, rigid patterns of function that limit and hamper our deepest healing resources and capacities.

THE SPECTRUM OF THERAPIES

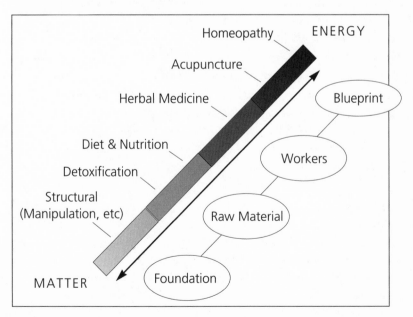

3. Health

Symptoms and Health

Health is much more than just an absence of symptoms, though this is the yardstick we usually use to judge our state of wellness. In fact, a healthy organism produces "symptoms" as part of its inherent ability to defend, adapt, respond, and improve itself. From a homeopathic point of view, every expression of life is a "symptom," though not necessarily an indication of "disease."

Health Defined

Health can be defined as having the internal capacity and freedom to experience and explore one's unique human potential and creativity.

PHYSICAL HEALTH is characterized by:

- Feeling dynamic, energetic, alive, vital, vibrant.
- Optimal metabolism of foods and nutrients, through the process of digestion, assimilation, and cellular respiration.
- The ability to adequately detoxify from cells, tissues, and organs.
- Optimal communication among all parts, so that the body and mind function as an integrated whole, not as fragmented elements.
- Freedom from the debilitating, weakening effects of chronic illness.
- The ability to respond appropriately and congruently to stress, toxins, or infectious processes, returning us to our previous state of health.

PSYCHOLOGICAL HEALTH is characterized by:

- An inner level of peace and calm or joy, not as a continual feeling, but as an internal *foundation* of our experience in the world.
- Confidence, assurance, and recognition of one's personal possibilities and potential and unconditional "OKayness."
- Motivation, interest, curiosity, and engagement with life.
- Courage, determination, and the many other qualities that express a fully individuated and mature state of emotional health.
- Freedom from debilitating anxiety, depression, states of anger and frustration, jealousy, and so on.
- Integration of our "dark side": hidden impulses, negativity, or motives that we have split off from and deny, yet act out *unconsciously*.
- Having non-dysfunctional, mutually beneficial relationships with others, and the capacity for tolerance, compassion, and love.

SPIRITUAL HEALTH is expressed by:
- An integration of intuition and intellect, vision and reason.
- Clarity of perception, free from habitual judgements or associations.
- A clear vision and central meaning to one's life, from which we derive our goals, our purpose and motivation, and our system of values.
- An ongoing search for deeper truth, meaning, and insight.
- A healthy development of one's sense of self. A lack of inner cohesion or congruence is one of the greatest problems challenging people today. Its flip side is the narcissistic, self-inflated, greedy, or selfish patterns that are a profound cause of illness on all levels today.

HEALTH IS INDIVIDUAL
- Though a generalized definition of health is important, it cannot be applied rigidly to real, individual people.
- The *experience* of health is as highly variable as our individual make-up and history, and our particular stage and process.
- Health is relative to what problems or deficits we have started with, and to how well we have adapted, changed, and improved our state.
- Our personal definition of "health" is related to our level of knowledge, and to what we understand about our potential capabilities.
- Based on the above ideals of wellness, very few of us can be considered completely "healthy." Though rare, it is yet what we strive for.
- *Homeopathy is capable of assisting the recovery and maintenance of health on any and all of these levels.*

THE SPECTRUM OF HEALTH

Health is not a static point, but a continuum, a spectrum through which we travel, as discussed below and in the accompanying chart.

(1) MEDIAN LEVEL
At any point in time, there is a level of functioning and feeling that we consider health. This *median level* is our normal state of vitality, our usual level of comfort or discomfort, our typical state of affairs.

(2) REDUCED LEVEL OF HEALTH
There is a lower level of health than our normal state, which we may enter only temporarily and rarely, or more frequently and intensely. When we drop down into this level, we call it illness.

(3) OPTIMAL LEVEL
There is an intensified level of physical and mental performance, and a sense of wellness that we aspire to, and occasionally experience.

a. Within the the range of the median level, there are fluctuations, having "good days" and "bad days," dependent on all kinds of variables.

b. There also are peak experiences, when we are lifted out of our normal level and feel elevated, a way we wish we could feel all the time. Sometimes this is just "how I used to feel when I was really well."

c. Illness occurs when we are overwhelmed by biological or psychological stresses and lose our adaptability and responsiveness. This should be a temporary healing crisis that returns us to full capacity.

d. Unfortunately, the tendency is for people to slip, gradually or dramatically, to a lower level, which eventually becomes the norm, with less vitality, more symptoms, and reduced function. Progressively falling to ever lower levels is characteristic of chronic, degenerative disease, and of much of what is mistakenly called "aging."

e. In any true improvement of health, we are shifting our median point, improving the level we call "normal" towards the optimal.

THE SPECTRUM OF HEALTH

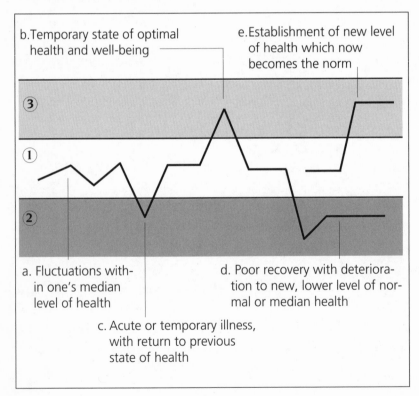

b. Temporary state of optimal health and well-being

e. Establishment of new level of health which now becomes the norm

a. Fluctuations within one's median level of health

d. Poor recovery with deterioration to new, lower level of normal or median health

c. Acute or temporary illness, with return to previous state of health

4. THE LIFE FORCE

BIOLOGICAL INTELLIGENCE

Even the most casual or cursory examination of the natural world impresses us with its rich complexity, extremely high degree of organization and co-ordination, and its ability to adapt and respond in inventive and creative ways. An inherent, intrinsic biological intelligence also co-ordinates every aspect of our physical life: digesting, breathing, heart pumping, clearing of wastes and toxins from the body, and the healing of tissue. The simple appreciation and respect for *life as intelligent, rather than mechanical*, is what dramatically differentiates traditional and holistic health care from contemporary medical thinking and therapy.

The concept of "life force" (prana, chi, dynamis) is the cornerstone of most systems of natural healing, and has been universally recognized and rediscovered throughout all times and cultures. This concept results in perceiving health, illness, and the possibility of cure in a more comprehensive way. The purpose of health care then becomes all about finding ways to access, reactivate, and work with inherent healing capacities. Though the term "life force" may seem antiquated, its meaning is based on observed facts and common sense. It is no more quasi-religious or mystical than seeing a tree grow from an acorn to a mighty oak. The immune, nervous, and hormonal systems are key components of the body's intelligent control and response systems.

ASPECTS OF THE LIFE FORCE

- *Intelligence*: The most obvious quality of the life force is intelligence. This is clearly expressed by the remarkable processes seen in nature: animals that return thousands of miles to the place of their birth; symbiotic relationships between insects and plants; and even the simple act of eating a carrot and turning it into human flesh!
- *Control*: We are familiar with the body's overall control systems, including the immune, nervous, and hormonal systems. The science of psychoneuroimmunology demonstrates that these systems function as a unified whole, with very intricate intercommunication. They also interface with our emotions and thoughts. Biological intelligence exerts its control through these systems but is not identical to them.
- *Energy*: Life force is part of, and expresses itself through, energy systems. The chakra system of ancient India and meridian system of acupuncture were early systems that investigated subtle functions of the life force.

- *Adaptability*: Life finds a way, and life forms adapt to the most harsh and inhospitable terrain, whether it is trees growing on the sheer face of a mountain, or flowers in an arid desert. Seemingly unlimited strategies and compensations allow the body to be extremely resourceful and adaptive to changes in climate, nutrition, and level of health.
- *Response-ability*: Apart from its long-term adaptive ability, an organism has the ability to respond to immediate changes in its environment.

DISEASE AND LIFE FORCE

The life force resides in the deepest core of the individual. In homeopathy, it is considered that all disease starts in the life force, and all disease affects the life force. In acute disease the biological intelligence responds dramatically, using intense means to push disease away from the center. Biological intelligence has as a priority protection of the most vital and important aspects of the individual. This hierarchy of tissues, organs, and psychological factors will be discussed in Topic 16.

STRONG VITALITY

In the young and in the healthy, there is an excess of energy, with optimal cellular metabolism and all organs at their biochemical and physiological peak. People with a good inheritance of vitality (a "robust constitution") will be able to have very acute, strong illnesses that do not linger. They also will respond dramatically to homeopathic medicines. Their symptoms will be vivid and clearly defined, as an expression of a strong, congruent life force.

INADEQUATE VITALITY

When vitality is low, resources are limited. The biological response systems may be inoperative or unavailable. Then even slight causes can overwhelm the compromised immune and nervous systems. Symptoms will be vague and unclear with the body unable to mount an adequate or meaningful response. Deep-acting homeopathics may be too demanding; these people require remedies that slowly rebuild the organism and the vitality.

RESPONSE TO MEDICINAL STIMULI

In natural medicine, it is the person that does all the healing, and medicines are simply catalysts for change. This also means that all healing takes place at the *expense* of the individual. Homeopathic remedies require a response from the life force. If an individual's resources are inadequate, this stimulus to change is useless, or may represent a stress on the organism, rather than a healing impetus.

5. SYMPTOMS

THE SECRET OF SYMPTOMS

An understanding of symptoms is at the very core of homeopathic principles and practice, yet homeopathy perceives symptoms in a radically different way than contemporary medicine. Modern medicine looks at illness as a "disease-entity," a self-existent thing that stalks our lives, waiting to pounce on unsuspecting victims. In this model, symptoms are seen as belonging *to the disease*, and so one "gets" the symptoms when one "has" the disease.

Homeopathy considers symptoms of illness as physiological, biological, and psychological *responses* or reactions to various causative factors. From this standpoint, symptoms *belong to people, not to diseases*. Though people have similar or typical reaction patterns, this still does not mean that their illnesses are external "entities" that implant their symptoms upon people. Causes of illness, including viruses, bacteria, injuries, nutritional deficiency, etc., also do not possess or confer symptoms. Thus, the point of homeopathy is to stimulate and assist natural healing responses, as expressed by symptoms. Conventional medicine seeks to remove offending symptoms (response mechanisms), since they are seen as synonymous with disease. But suppressing symptoms without removing causes or strengthening the body merely weakens the health and promotes future problems; it is based on a misperception of how biological systems actually work.

SYMPTOM INDIVIDUALITY

Though people share similar response patterns to a specific stimulus, the similarity is only superficial. No two symptomatic responses are exactly identical. Thus in any disease category there are dozens or even hundreds of possible symptom patterns expressed by different individuals. As a result there can be hundreds of possible remedies for a particular disease or syndrome.

SYMPTOMS ARE POSITIVE-TENDING

As a natural biological response to an irritating cause, symptoms are inherently *positive or health promoting* attempts by the body and mind to cure itself. It is the central goal of every organism to survive and flourish, and all symptoms produced by the body must be considered adaptive measures, attempts to deal successfully with the causes of illness.

SYMPTOMS ARE MEANINGFUL

As positive responses, each symptom is *meaningful* and purposeful. Symptoms are an extremely accurate language of body, mind, and spirit. The particular style of symptoms expressed by a person also demonstrates their biological and psychological type, e.g. their *constitution*. Just as we can know a person by their quality of speech, their dress, habits and actions, so do external symptoms reveal the "inner person."

PROGRESSION OF SYMPTOMS

Symptoms and illness progress from the level of *sensation*, to become *functional* disturbances, and finally *pathological* or cellular disease. The disturbance in a person's health first takes place on an intangible, subtle energetic level, the level of biological intelligence. Subjective symptoms, subtle experiences of imbalance, discomfort, or unusual sensations occur long before any other evidence of illness.

If causes continue to act, functional changes eventually occur, resulting in a disturbance of normal physiology, e.g., cramps, nasal discharge, etc. If these causes are invasive or persistent enough, eventually chemical and finally cellular changes will follow, resulting in pathology. Unfortunately, it is only at this last stage of the progression of illness that medical diagnostics can definitively make a particular diagnosis! With increased pathology, individualized symptoms and sensations may diminish, leaving the case more "generic" and difficult to treat from a homeopathic point of view.

TYPES OF SYMPTOMS

Though all symptoms are positive, adaptive responses of our biological intelligence, all symptoms are not created equal! Some symptoms are *acute responses* to intense toxic, infective, or stressful impacts. These physiological reactions are designed to eradicate, neutralize, or assimilate these causative factors, and return the organism to normal. Symptoms also may be *chronic* and part of a long-term adaptive trend, a holding pattern that prevents a more rapid acceleration of disease, but does not allow for real cure or removal of causes. The organism may have lost its capacity to do so, or may be unable to access these internal resources.

Homeopathic remedies can help resolve the acute symptoms produced by the body, and convert chronic illness to acute or healing reactions. Under the influence of the correct homeopathic remedy, the person —body and mind — may be stimulated to undergo a healing crisis, in which the body's reactivated defense mechanisms are rallied to throw off ongoing chronic causes and patterns of disease. These healing symptoms are often identical to symptoms experienced previously by the individual, during an earlier stage of the illness.

Generation of Symptoms

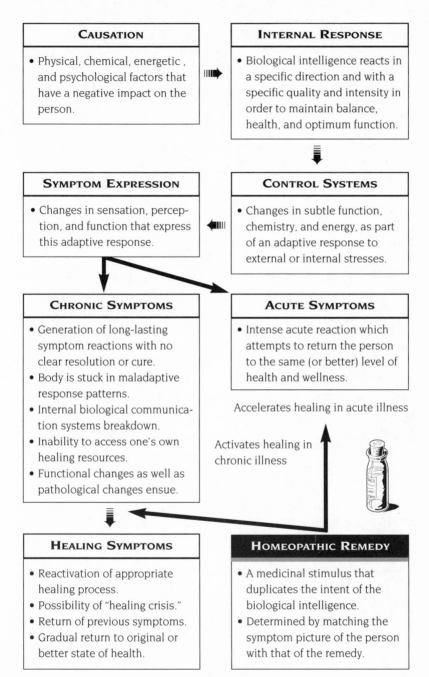

CAUSATION

- Physical, chemical, energetic , and psychological factors that have a negative impact on the person.

INTERNAL RESPONSE

- Biological intelligence reacts in a specific direction and with a specific quality and intensity in order to maintain balance, health, and optimum function.

SYMPTOM EXPRESSION

- Changes in sensation, perception, and function that express this adaptive response.

CONTROL SYSTEMS

- Changes in subtle function, chemistry, and energy, as part of an adaptive response to external or internal stresses.

CHRONIC SYMPTOMS

- Generation of long-lasting symptom reactions with no clear resolution or cure.
- Body is stuck in maladaptive response patterns.
- Internal biological communication systems breakdown.
- Inability to access one's own healing resources.
- Functional changes as well as pathological changes ensue.

ACUTE SYMPTOMS

- Intense acute reaction which attempts to return the person to the same (or better) level of health and wellness.

Accelerates healing in acute illness

Activates healing in chronic illness

HEALING SYMPTOMS

- Reactivation of appropriate healing process.
- Possibility of "healing crisis."
- Return of previous symptoms.
- Gradual return to original or better state of health.

HOMEOPATHIC REMEDY

- A medicinal stimulus that duplicates the intent of the biological intelligence.
- Determined by matching the symptom picture of the person with that of the remedy.

SYMPTOMS AS THE BASIS OF REMEDIES

Since symptoms express the direction and force of the healing reaction, they are an accurate guide to determining and assisting the biological and psychological attempts at healing. The *form* and *nature* of symptoms contain all the information required to *stimulate* and *emulate* the activity of biological intelligence, which is actively working to create a healthy individual. A homeopath, using these symptoms as a guide, prescribes a *medicine* that will work to achieve that stimulation.

PROVINGS

In order to prescribe such a remedy, a homeopath needs to know exactly how a medicine will work on the body. The scientific research technique used by homeopaths to arrive at this knowledge is known as a *proving*. Healthy individuals are given repeated doses of a homeopathic medicine over a period of time, until it elicits symptoms that were not there before. Recording all these subjective symptom responses, a very detailed and accurate *remedy picture* is built up. Historical use, accidental poisonings, and clinical results over the last 200 years confirm and expand our understanding of the remedies.

- By *saturating the person* with the biological and biochemical information inherent in a specific natural substance and seeing how they respond, the individual become a "sounding board," for the direction and force of the healing properties within the remedy. This process is neither dangerous or toxic for the participants, nor does it rely on animal research.
- The detailed remedy picture becomes the basis of the homeopathic materia medica, the remedies used to treat all manner of human illness.
- We then know exactly in what way a remedy influences a person. Since symptoms of illness express the body's self-healing attempts, the correct remedy will merely *reinforce this activity*, accelerating healing.

SYMPTOMS OF LIFE

Shifting one's view of symptoms from being wholly negative phenomena to being an expression of one's own intelligence has profound consequences. Instead of trying, at all costs, to suppress symptoms, they are seen as important messengers and guides towards healing. This dramatically changes our approach to our own and other people's illness. Symptoms become friend instead of foe. On the other hand, suppression of symptoms inevitably has very negative consequences. Finally, all symptoms are a *language* that articulates our deepest humanness and vibrancy as both a biological organism and as a spiritual being. The connotation of fear and loathing that has been created around symptoms is itself a source of psychological and physical illness.

6. MODALITIES

ESSENTIAL MODIFIERS OF SYMPTOMS

Modalities are factors that make any particular symptom better or worse. These are crucial to an accurate homeopathic prescription. Though the physiological meaning of modalities may at times be obscure or seem to have no logic, they are extremely important for the selection of the correct homeopathic remedy. For a *medical* diagnosis modalities are nothing; for a *homeopathic* diagnosis they are everything. They clarify the symptom language of the body. A person in suffering will naturally know what makes him / her feel better or worse, even though they may have not really *thought* about it.

Modalities must be *clear* and *definite* in order to be useful guides. There are many modalities, but they can be easily put into categories. For every symptom, modalities should be looked for in each category.

1. TIME: of the day, week, month, season, phases of the moon, regularity, recurrence, periodicity (every three days, etc.), during menses, sunrise.
2. TEMPERATURE: hot or cold environment, winds, air, bathing, hot or cold applications, going from hot to cold or vice versa, etc.
3. ENVIRONMENT: damp and rain, foggy, overcast or clear, seashore, mountain air, high elevations, changes in barometric pressure, etc.
4. POSITION: posture, sitting, lying, standing, lying on one side or the other, on the painful or painless side, etc.
5. MOTION: worse or better from movement, gentle or vigorous exertion, after rest, from initial movement, stretching, bending, after prolonged use, bending double, rising up, ascending or descending, etc.
6. BODY ACTIVITY: talking, eating, defecating, sneezing, urinating, perspiring, sexual activity, travelling, drinking, after sleeping or a nap, etc.
7. SENSORY: odors, touch, noise, music, light, pressure, jarring, etc.
8. PSYCHOLOGICAL: from excitement, fear, loss or grief, suppressed emotions, overwork or overstudy, when thinking of one's complaint.

Additionally, LOCATIONS may be included as part of modalities, e.g. tending to occur on the left or right side, from above down, etc. The effects of SPECIFIC FOODS may also be listed with modalities, including aggravations from coffee, sugar, alcohol, cold water, etc. Modality categories and some typical examples are shown on the next page.

MODALITIES

TIME
- Specific time or period of day
- Day vs. night
- Weekly, monthly
- Season
- Menses
- Recurring

MOTION
- Initial motion
- Rest
- Exertion
- Gentle motion
- Walking, lifting
- Rising up
- Stretching

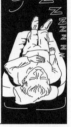

TEMPERATURE
- Heat
  of sun, bed, room
- Cold
  air, water, wind
- Hot compresses
- Cold bathing
- Change of temp.

BODY ACTIVITY
- Eating / Drinking
- Urinating
- Defecation
- Sleep
- Coughing
- Yawning
- Sexual activity

WEATHER
- Damp
  damp & cold
  hot & humid
- Sunny / Foggy
- Storms
- Weather changes
- Clear / Overcast

SENSORY
- Touch
- Pressure
- Noise
- Music
- Light
- Odors

POSITION
- Lying, standing
- Sitting
- Stooping
- Stretched out
- Doubled up
- Right or left side
- Stiff or limp

PSYCHOLOGICAL
- Overstudy
- When busy
- Excitement
- Anger
- Worry
- Thinking about it

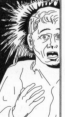

7. DISEASE

DISEASE REDEFINED

Symptoms of "disease" are actually our natural, positive-tending responses to some kind of negative stimuli, some factor or cause that we experience as a threat or potential danger. Disease symptoms, if successful, restore us to balance and a full state of health. Illness can be looked at as the interplay of three factors or variables:

1. Causes   2. Symptom Responses   3 Reaction Patterns.

Having discussed Symptoms in Topic 5, this section looks at causes from the homeopathic point of view. Reaction patterns are discussed briefly at the end of this section and in Topic 16.

THE NATURE OF CAUSES

- Disease is rarely due to a single, independent cause. In fact it is *multi-causal*: many varied and different influences add together or *summate* to eventually overwhelm the individual and create illness.
- Causes may be external or internal factors, recent or very remote, physical or psychological. What matters is how deep an impact they have made on our being and how they affect the life force.
- There is a natural hierarchy of causes, yet at any point in time the most intense, limiting factor assumes greatest importance for an individual.
- Many causes of illness are not chemical or material. Old injuries, toxic drugs, emotional trauma, past illness; all these can leave an energetic pattern or *imprint* that exists indefinitely, and continues to erode the health and well-being of a person.
- Since these imprints or patterns exist on an energetic or information level, homeopathy is the ultimate tool for neutralizing them.
- If actual physical residues do remain, these can be eliminated when remedies mobilize the immune system and detoxification pathways.

CAUSES AND MODALITIES

- Causes should not be confused with modalities, though the factor itself — for example, dampness — can be identical.
- Dampness is a *modality* when it makes an *existing* condition better or worse. If dampness, experienced over a period of time, permanently alters the person's health, it has become a causative factor.
- A modality can also initiate an episode of a particular existing illness, such as bringing on a headache, or an attack of arthritis. In a strict sense this could be termed a *precipitating cause*.

CATEGORIES OF CAUSES

The accompanying "Hierarchy of Causes" diagram shows the categories of causes that impact our health, as outlined below:

ENVIRONMENTAL CAUSES

• Though they are almost completely ignored in contemporary medicine, environmental causes have always been considered important in traditional health systems, such as Chinese Medicine.
• Homeopathic remedies include such causes within their symptom picture, including "rheumatism after exposure to damp weather," the effects of living or working in damp or cold places, or getting chilled.

STRUCTURAL CAUSES

• Many musculoskeletal remedies are appropriate for problems "after an injury in the remote past," or at the site of an old strain, and so on.
• Structural causes include injuries, sprains, repeated strains, fractures, surgical procedures, overexertion, or prolonged lifting activity.
• Postural causes include sedentary habits, sitting bent over, etc. Though postural traits are sometimes included in the constitutional description of remedies, much more research is needed in this area.

TOXIC CAUSES

• Toxicity is well known to modern medicine, though usually only the immediate or obvious effects of toxins are taken in account. Toxic causes include a wide range of categories including the following:
  — *Chemicals*: the short- and long-term effects of heavy metals, industrial pollutants in the air and water, food additives, pesticides, etc.
  — *Drugs*: cumulative toxic and damaging effects of prescription and non-prescription drugs, and the potential residual effects of vaccines.
  — *Metabolic by-products*: toxins formed through normal metabolism, and retained in the tissues, toxic build up in the liver, colon, etc.
  — *Allergens*: dietary and airborne allergens and chemical sensitivities.

INFECTIOUS CAUSES

  — *Microbes*: bacteria, viruses, parasites; lingering effects or poor recovery from past illnesses, including venereal diseases.
  — *Suppression* of acute illness has considerable negative impact, driving toxins deeper and thwarting the body's attempts to detoxify tissues.

  Note: There are remedies appropriate to illnesses caused by particular toxins, microbes, drugs, or heavy metals, and these remedies also often have the ability to antidote that factor, helping eliminate any residues from the body. More research in this area will provide better tools for surviving and staying well in today's polluted world.

NUTRITIONAL CAUSES

Nutrient deficiencies and imbalances contribute significantly to the development of degenerative disease, and though beyond the scope of this book, the impact of nutrition on musculoskeletal health is profound. However, homeopathy plays an important role in dealing with nutritional causes of illness, because remedies can dramatically improve the digestion, assimilation, and delivery of nutrients to the tissues, helping the body metabolize and utilized them more efficiently.

PSYCHOLOGICAL CAUSES

An appreciation of the intimate relationship between mind and body is central to homeopathy, and psychological factors are high in the hierarchy of causes. There are many remedies for the short- or long-term effects of an emotional shock, upset, grief, loss, fit of anger or fright. Suppressed or unexpressed feelings can be important factors in the genesis of disease and numerous remedies directly address these hidden, unresolved emotional experiences.

CONSTITUTION

We have inherent predispositions and tendencies towards specific illnesses, pathology, locations, and physical and mental symptoms. Central to the development and progress of chronic illness, acquired or genetic patterns of predisposition (termed *miasms* in homeopathy) can be neutralized or eradicated by deep-acting constitutional remedies.

SUPPRESSION

Suppression creates disease and accelerates existing illness, driving it deeper into the system. This includes suppression of natural discharges (such as perspiration, nasal discharges, or menses), and suppression of illness (such as skin disease, venereal disease, or fever).

DISEASE AS FIXATION

Our body and mind respond to factors which can make us ill. If this response is *appropriate*, and the causes are something we can handle, we will produce internal changes and a symptom picture that effectively deals with the problem. Unfortunately, due to heredity, experience, past illness, and a host of other factors, we begin to lose our reactive capacity, even at an early age. The body / mind response to stressors becomes mechanical instead of adaptive, and we fail to draw on our wider resources and capabilities. *Maladaptive response patterns* develop, or we become stuck or fixated into a limited, locked-in reaction pattern. Homeopathy is the primary therapy for dissolving fixations, allowing inherent deep-level patterns of wellness to reinstate themselves.

THE HIERARCHY OF CAUSES

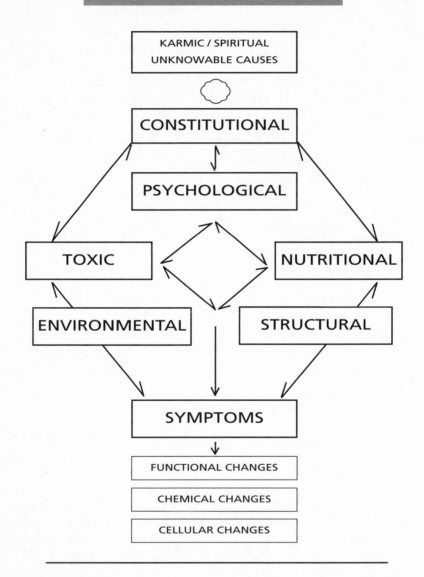

This diagram shows the categories and relative importance of different levels of cause. These causes are *interdependent* and mutually influence each other, as shown by the *two-way arrows*.

Ultimately the most important causes are the ones that are limiting the person the most, whatever their level might be.

8. CURE

HOMEOPATHIC CURE

The effect of giving a homeopathic medicine should be to:
• Initiate healing responses when they are sluggish or inadequate.
• Assist the body's ongoing attempts at self-healing and the *inherent biological processes* of detoxification, nutrition, and tissue regeneration.
• Re-establish communication between the parts and the whole.
• Remove blockages or hindrances to curative forces.
• Free the body from fixed patterns and locked-in modes of functioning which keep it from accessing its full capacities and resources.
• Restore the ability to live a full and creative life.
• Gently provide stimulus to the body/mind healing process, rather than forcing a reaction in an invasive, aggressive manner.

LEVELS OF CURE

SYMPTOMS

Symptoms inevitably cause suffering, weaken the individual, and interfere with the normal activity and freedom of body and mind. Homeopathy seeks to resolve symptoms (not suppress them) by helping the body remove the internal *causes* of disease and strengthen the defense system and adaptive capabilities of mind and body.

FUNCTION

Functional disturbances can be either an exaggeration of normal function (cramps) or intense physiological reactions, such as inflammation or fever. Though they cause only minimal tissue damage, these disturbances can be extremely debilitating and cause significant suffering. Functional problems are usually capable of complete cure, returning the body to its original capacities and restores normal function.

STRUCTURE

Pathological change occurs when there is an alteration of cells, tissues, and the actual structure of the body. With expert homeopathic care the progression of a destructive illness may be slowed or arrested altogether, and further damage prevented. Depending on the organ and type of tissue involved, and the nature of the disease, pathological change may be partly reversible, including, for example, the dissolving of internal adhesions and scar tissue, and the shrinking of benign growths and tumors.

SUSCEPTIBILITY

The deepest underlying causes of disease, from the homeopathic point of view, are specific *patterns of susceptibility* (miasms) which lead, inexorably, towards degenerative conditions. Whether these inherent weaknesses are genetic or acquired,they can be diminished, made latent, or even eradicated with expert homeopathic treatment. Ultimately this translates into longer life, free from the spectre of chronic disease in general, as attested to by many historical homeopaths, who lived to a very ripe and healthy old age! Homeopathy is a form of *preventive medicine* par excellence!

LEVEL OF HEALTH

When a variety of significant causes are removed by homeopathic remedies, the metabolic, neurological, hormonal, and immune functions regain their potential for optimal functioning. Thus we change the basic *level of health* of the person.

PSYCHOLOGICAL HEALING

Improvement in mental functioning, including concentration, memory, and clarity is important evidence that a constitutional remedy is working, regardless of the nature of the chief complaint. Homeopathy provides curative effects for acute and chronic emotional disturbances, including the full range of anger and irritability, anxiety and fear, or grief and depression. In a general way, curative reactions bring about an increase in psychological health, improving self-confidence and motivation, and promoting an attitude of optimism and clarity of purpose.

TRANSPERSONAL HEALING

Homeopathy can assist the deepest levels of personal growth and integration, helping an individual to access his or her innermost core of values, insight, and sense of presence.

PALLIATION

In cases where profound cure and reversal of existing disease is not possible, homeopathy can still provide invaluable help in reducing symptoms and providing increased energy, improving the general level of well-being. It is not always advisable or appropriate to dig deeply into the constitution if age and pathology warrant against it.

SUPPRESSION

• Suppression of pain, inflammation, or troubling symptoms is the basis of the mainstream attitude towards health and disease. This viewpoint treats illness and symptoms as enemies to be eliminated, repressed, or destroyed. By attacking a symptom, one supposedly destroys the disease to which it belongs. Since symptoms actually *belong to the person*, this approach has, unfortunately, led to a system that does not work with the body, but against it, using toxic and often harmful medicines.

Suppression and palliation may have their place (such as pain-killers), as long as this is not erroneously confused with or described as cure. However, *suppression is not synonymous with cure* and removal of symptoms without removing the *causes* of the illness, has a long-term negative impact on the health. Suppression *inevitably* results in deeper, more invasive disease states later on, even though this commonly occurs in areas of the body seemingly unrelated to the original condition.

PROGNOSIS

The prognosis of a condition, or the possible extent of cure, depends on a complex mixture of factors, some of which are listed below:
— Duration of the illness
— Nature of the disease or condition
— Nature of the person: their age, vitality, susceptibilities
— Specific location or tissues involved
— Degree of pathological tissue change that has already occurred
— Phase of illness, i.e. whether acute, chronic or advanced
— Previous suppressive treatment
— Ongoing causes (environmental toxins, poor nutrition, stress, etc.)
— Oversensitivity or hyperactivity of the immune system
— Past history of illness, and if recovered from adequately
— Family history and tendencies
— Psychological blocks or ongoing conflicts which complicate cure
— Openness to change, or resistance to change on various levels
— The prescriber's skill, experience, and training

CURABILITY

There are certain indicators that cure will be difficult, because the body cannot mount a congruent and cohesive defense or response:
• Remedies may work only a short time, and then cease to be useful.
• Symptoms are chaotic or make little sense, homeopathically.
• There is a *lack* of symptoms or of modalities in a clearly sick individual, indicating a poorly reactive immune system.
• Extreme mental and physical rigidity may be an obstacle to cure, or may be the most important symptom for prescribing a curative remedy.
• In many so-called "incurable" patients, revitalizing remedies can be used to build up strength and vitality. Local remedies and low potencies can gradually change the state of pathology.

9. HOMEOPATHIC REMEDIES

SOURCES

- Remedies are generally derived from the natural realms of plant, mineral, and animal. Approximately 70% of remedies are of herbal or plant origin, though many of the deepest-acting remedies are minerals.
- Remedies may derive from healing substances (Marigold flowers), neutral substances (table salt), or toxic substances (Arsenic).
- Through the homeopathic pharmaceutical process, they all become powerful and deep-acting medicines.
- If a remedy is a healing herb in its native state, it retains many of its healing indications when in homeopathic form (Calendula flowers).
- Poisonous substances often have curative effects which are *opposite* to the toxic effect of taking a material dose (Arsenic causes diarrhea but homeopathic Arsenicum cures diarrhea).
- *Nosodes* are a class of remedies made from microorganisms or disease substances. Like other homeopathic remedies they are prescribed based on their total symptom picture, not just for a bacterial disease.
- Remedies have been prepared from *non-material sources*, such as moonlight, musical frequencies, electricity, and the south pole of a magnet.

ENERGY MEDICINE

All substances have a specific vibrational pattern, not unlike the frequencies of a radio wave or sound wave, but of a far more subtle and complex nature. Just as a substance is *unique* in its chemical and physical structure, it is unique in its vibrational or energetic make-up. Physicists now believe that these patterns or "morphogenic fields" precede and determine the chemical and physical structure of matter — a view that is consistent with many ancient healing systems.

The homeopathic pharmacological process is capable of extracting the inherent pattern or energy blueprint from gross material substances. Remedies are "dynamized" or "potentized," becoming an increasingly subtle energetic force, capable of deep therapeutic action. Though the ides of "bioenergy" is consistent with the knowledge of contemporary physics, the biological sciences have yet to integrate this idea. A technology to accurately measure or differentiate the energy "fingerprint" of a particular flower, mineral, or living creature does not exist yet; full scientific validation of homeopathy may have to await the creation of a device sensitive enough to measure bioenergetic patterns.

THE INFINITESIMAL DOSE

- The infinitesimal or microdose is a unique contribution of homeopathy to the art of healing, and is one of its most controversial aspects. Extracting the energy pattern described earlier is accomplished by a process of dilution and succession in a mathematical series. This is fully explained in many homeopathic books and is summarized in the accompanying diagram. Less of the original substance means a deeper effect, as a remedy becomes increasingly more energetic and less material: the higher the number of dilutions, the stronger and deeper the remedy acts.
- Topic 14 discusses the relative merits of using "high" or "low" potencies.

REMEDY PREPARATION

- Plants, generally still fresh, are made into alcoholic extracts or tinctures (mother tinctures). Non-soluble minerals or metals are first ground down with milk sugar as the diluting agent. These are called triturations.
- Remedies are made by a series of dilutions, either on the scale of 1 part of original substance to 9 parts of alcohol or water, or 1 part to 99.
- This creates either the decimal scale ("x"), or the centesimal scale ("c").
- Potencies are named according to the number of times they have been diluted and shaken up (*succussed*) in the x or c scale. (e.g. 6x, 30c, 200c).
- In all probability, remedies beyond the 12c or 24x level contain *no atoms or molecules* of the original substance: they are purely "energy medicine."
- The other component of remedy-making is succussion, a process whereby the remedy is shaken vigorously between each sequence of dilution.
- This process helps release the energetic essence of the substance.
- These successive steps are termed potencies or dilutions.
- The dynamized remedies are finally put into a carrier substance, usually sugar pellets but sometimes tablets, tiny granules, or liquid drops.
- The administration and care of remedies is the subject of Topic 15.

NON-TOXICITY

The first tenet of Hippocrates, the so-called father of medicine, was "Above all, do no harm." Homeopathic medicines have no inherent toxicity and as a result have no side effects. Conversely, many medical drugs only treat symptoms while producing many unwanted effects. For example, anti-inflammatory drugs used for arthritis (Aspirin, Motrin, and Naprosyn) actually accelerate the deterioration of joint cartilage.

Homeopathic remedies do, however, cause reactions that can occasionally be intense. These are part of the healing process, rather than side-effects, and are sometimes necessary in order to return the person to health. As powerful healing agents, homeopathic medicines must be used with care and precision.

REMEDY PREPARATION

① ORIGINAL SUBSTANCE

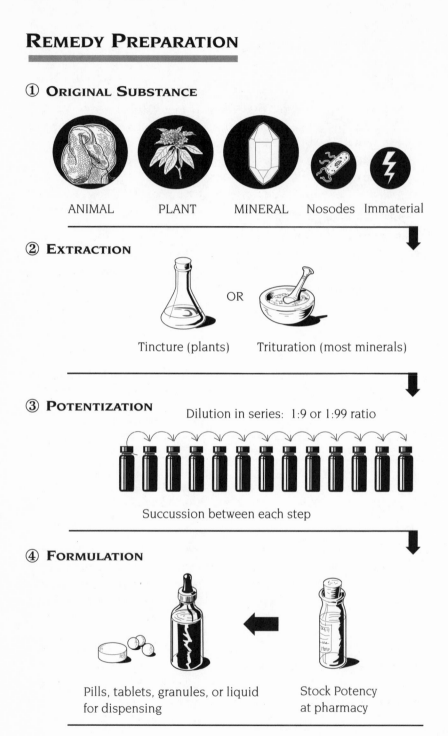

ANIMAL   PLANT   MINERAL   Nosodes   Immaterial

② EXTRACTION

OR

Tincture (plants)   Triturition (most minerals)

③ POTENTIZATION

Dilution in series: 1:9 or 1:99 ratio

Succussion between each step

④ FORMULATION

Pills, tablets, granules, or liquid   Stock Potency
for dispensing   at pharmacy

10. THE PRINCIPLE OF SIMILARS

LIKE CURES LIKE

The so-called "Principle of Similars" is the cornerstone of homeopathy and expresses a profound truth about how biological and psychological healing really work. Any substance will cause certain symptoms when given in excess; yet this same substance will cure those very symptoms when given to a sick person. This is based on the fact that symptoms are an expression of the internal process of self-healing rather that an expression of a disease per se. The process of homeopathic remedy selection helps clarify the Principle of Similars.

First a detailed *symptom picture of the person* is obtained through taking a survey of all symptoms and modalities during the homeopathic case history. A detailed *symptom picture of a remedy* is available to us through research provings and our homeopathic materia medica. By matching the remedy picture with the person's symptom picture, we are matching the *direction and force* of the body's own healing reaction with the reaction stimulated by the remedy. We are emulating and reinforcing the activity of biological intelligence, assisting the organism in a direction that it is already attempting to move, with changes that it is already attempting to make.

We would *not need* to match the symptoms of person and remedy if we had another way of discovering exactly what substance would promote the healing forces of an individual. As it is, the language of symptoms is an accurate guide to gauge the nature and form of the internal healing process. Optimally, the *potency* or strength of the remedy should match the depth of the illness; its relative material or energetic level.

THE PRINCIPLE OF OPPOSITES

Conventional drugs are called *allopathic*, as opposed to homeopathic. Generally they reduce symptoms by interfering with the body's physiological or reactive processes, rather than assisting the inherent self-corrective mechanisms. Though necessary at times, medicines which remove symptoms without removing causes or strengthening organs or tissues ultimately reduce health. Invasive and toxic treatments disrupt the body and undermine biological intelligence and integrity, contributing to the epidemic immune system failure we are witnessing today. Like a muscle, if not allowed to exercise freely this intelligent biological response system will atrophy, losing its ability to meet daily challenges.

ACTIONS OF SIMILAR MEDICINES

Hahnemann, the developer of homeopathy, explained the action of remedies as a "displacement" phenomenon, whereby a stronger artificial remedy-disease displaces the real illness. When the symptoms of this artificial, remedy-induced syndrome evaporate, the person is left free of both it and the original sickness. From a physiological standpoint, we can say that we are stimulating and reinforcing the action of the immune system and other control mechanisms in responding to negative biological influences. From the viewpoint of energy medicine, we are supplying a specific vibrational frequency or pattern that neutralizes the disease frequency, while reinforcing our own bioenergy system. We are also giving the body and mind *information* about the symptom response it is undergoing (its so-called disease).

If disease is considered the result of fixed or limited patterns of response, the remedy acts as a mirror-image, showing the body the pattern in which it is stuck or fixated. With this information, the body can move out of a particular limited reaction pattern and use its larger resources and possibilities. In this way homeopathy supports and strengthens the intelligent control systems of the body. Whatever the final mechanism of action of a homeopathic remedy, in the final analysis, the modus operandi is simply to match the *symptoms* of the remedy with the *symptoms* of the patient.

TYPES OF SIMILARITY

There are different degrees and levels of "similarity" between the remedy and the person:

- A remedy may match only the mental symptoms of a person.
- It may only correspond to the local or acute symptoms experienced in a particular part of the body.
- A remedy may match the location or type of tissue involved, the physiological process taking place, or the type of disease pathology.
- It may match the entire metabolism, physical type, and psychological profile of the individual.
- The most profound-acting remedy will be the one that most clearly matches the utmost core of the individual, their *essence* or archetype.
- Nevertheless, because of the limited number of remedies available to us, the many layers of obstacles to cure, and the state of our health, the perfect remedy may not always be available. It may be necessary to give a series of remedies over time, in order to uncover ever deeper layers.
- More information on types of similarities and different ways of prescribing is given in Topics 12 and 13.

THE PRINCIPLE OF SIMILARS

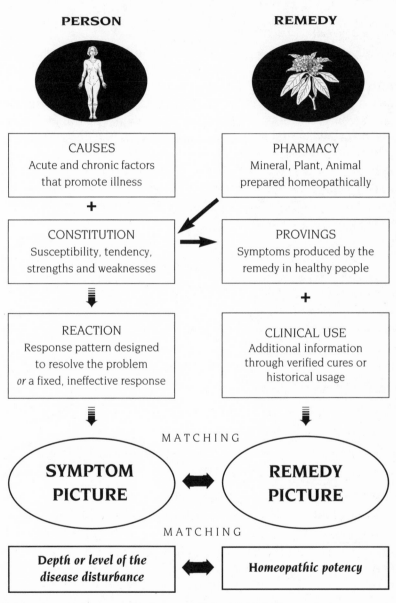

PERSON   **REMEDY**

CAUSES
Acute and chronic factors
that promote illness

PHARMACY
Mineral, Plant, Animal
prepared homeopathically

+

CONSTITUTION
Susceptibility, tendency,
strengths and weaknesses

PROVINGS
Symptoms produced by the
remedy in healthy people

+

REACTION
Response pattern designed
to resolve the problem
or a fixed, ineffective response

CLINICAL USE
Additional information
through verified cures or
historical usage

MATCHING

SYMPTOM PICTURE ⬌ **REMEDY PICTURE**

MATCHING

Depth or level of the disease disturbance ⬌ *Homeopathic potency*

If there is a perfect match, the remedy is the "Similimum."
If it only matches in part, but not at the core, it is a "similar" remedy.

11. CASE HISTORY

HOMEOPATHIC DIAGNOSIS

In homeopathy there are two diagnoses. The first is the diagnosis of the condition. The second "diagnosis" is the name of the remedy that will cure the condition — and the person who has it. In homeopathy, the name of the disease points one towards a class or group of remedies that are usually effective in treating this condition. But because there are many different homeopathic remedies possible for any one condition, the *final* choice of a remedy is based on the unique *subjective symptoms* and reactions that distinguish one person from another. On the other hand, conventional medical therapy tends to be general or *generic*, while homeopathy individualizes, focusing on the *person* with his or her own unique requirements.

HOMEOPATHIC PERCEPTION:

If homeopathic prescribing is based on "similarity" — finding a remedy picture that matches the symptom picture of the patient — the crux of the matter becomes deciding *which symptoms are to be matched.* A person's symptoms are not of equal value but exist in a hierarchy, a relative scale of importance in their meaning and depth. Perceiving "what is to be cured in an illness and in the person" is the core of prescribing and the most difficult skill to acquire in homeopathy.

VALUE OF SYMPTOMS

The case history, and not the laboratory, is the primary tool of homeopathy in determining what remedy is needed to heal a person. There is much to learn about how to elicit accurate and meaningful symptoms in homeopathy. For our purpose, some basic guidelines for assessing the importance of symptoms are outlined below.

CLARITY, INTENSITY, PECULIARITY

To gauge the value of a specific symptom, three factors are considered:
- *Clarity*: Vivid, well-defined symptoms are more important to the body than vague complaints. This includes the presence of clear modalities.
- *Intensity*: Intensity indicates the degree to which the symptom limits function or debilitates the person, physically or mentally.
- *Peculiarity*: The more atypical, rare, or unusual a symptom or reaction is, the more it relates to only a small or unique group of remedies.

- All symptoms can be classified on a scale of one to three, three being the most intense, clear, or rare, and having importance as regards location, depth of tissue, whether it is a generalized or local symptom, etc.

CHIEF COMPLAINTS

"Chief complaints" are the symptoms which are the person's greatest concerns and which they perceive as causing the most limitation. This may or may not be the most important problem. A person may not appreciate the deep-seated roots of a condition, and focus only on eliminating superficial, irritating symptoms, not essential causes.

ASSOCIATED SYMPTOMS

Called "concomitant symptoms" in homeopathy, these symptoms occur simultaneously with the main problem. They are important, whether or not they seem to make logical or anatomical sense.

CHRONOLOGY

Illness is not static, and the *onset* and *course* of illness can be decisive in finding the remedy which matches the progress of the illness. The *past history* acts as a guide to recognizing the emergence of previous symptoms during the course of cure. Our current illness is *always* related to our entire history of illness, problems, and stresses.

KEYNOTES

Keynotes are symptoms that are intense and definite, thus serving as a rapid key to a small and select group of remedies. Keynotes can also serve as *eliminating symptoms* — those that eliminate a whole range of remedies that do not possess this symptom. This method of prescribing requires a very firm grasp of the materia medica. Traditionally three *keynotes* are sought to confirm a remedy (like sitting on a three-legged stool). Each remedy has its own characteristic keynote symptoms.

SPECIFIC MUSCULOSKELETAL SYMPTOMS

In musculoskeletal conditions, certain *types of symptoms* are common and form the basis of a useful case history. The Materia Medica section of this book describes remedies according to this plan, describing pain, location, and associated symptoms or sensations.

PAIN

- *Definition:* Though often difficult for people to describe, the specific quality, intensity, and nature of the pain have important homeopathic diagnostic value. Condition Chart 1 may be used as a visual guide to help clarify and articulate the painful sensations.

SENSATIONS

- *Definition*: Other sensations may accompany the pain or predominate.
- Some of the most common musculoskeletal sensations include stiffness, tightness, constriction, numbness, formication (crawling), burning, heaviness, and weakness.
- Sensations should also be qualified and rounded out with their specific modalities, locations, and associated symptoms.
- Condition Chart 2 visually summarizes these many sensations.

LOCATION

- *Definition*: This includes the specific tissues, organs, and areas that are involved, both as described by the person and their actual anatomical location. Included is *radiation* or *extension*, i.e., the referral of pain or other sensations from the original site to another area.

ASSOCIATED SYMPTOMS

- *Definition*: Associated symptoms, such as the sensations described above, may appear along with the pain or may overshadow it. Symptoms in other organs or parts of the body may also be associated with the main complaint, occurring at the same time or alternating with it.
- Examples include restlessness, nausea or vomiting, headache (if not the primary complaint), faintness, emotional symptoms, skin eruptions, perspiration, and temperature alterations (feelings of heat or cold, locally or generally).

HISTORY OF THE PROBLEM

- *Definition*: The onset and course of illness, how long it has existed, and whether it has improved or deteriorated are all relevant to finding a remedy that matches the rhythm and progression of the condition.

CAUSATION

- *Definition*: If the condition or pain has a known cause, this can be extremely important to the selection of the correct remedy. A *remote cause* can be a single event, such as a fall or injury, or a prolonged stress, such as living in a damp climate for years. *Immediate causes*, such as bad weather, may also be important, since they trigger an attack of the illness.

MODALITIES

- For the musculoskeletal system, modalities of activity and position are particularly important, along with weather, temperature of the environment, local heat or cold, and time of day.
- The sample questionnaire that follows can be copied and used as a basic guide and outline for musculoskeletal case-taking.

MUSCULOSKELETAL QUESTIONNAIRE

- Answer the questions in the spaces below or use a separate page.
- In homeopathy, all symptoms are important, even if they are unusual, illogical, or don't seem related to your main complaint.
- Indicate the importance of each symptom you describe:
- <u>One underline</u> means the symptom is present, but not too serious.
- <u>Two underlines</u> means that the symptom is very clear and intense.
- <u>Three underlines</u> is for extremely intense, vivid, or serious symptoms.

What is your MAIN COMPLAINT?

_____

WHERE exactly is the pain or problem?

_____

What is the PAIN or main complaint like?

_____

Is there anything specific that BRINGS IT ON?

_____

How LONG does it last?

_____

If it is not constant, how does it BEGIN and END?

_____

Do you experience STIFFNESS? Describe where and when.

_____

Are you RESTLESS or do you desire to be STILL with the pain?

_____

Are there other symptoms or SENSATIONS in your joints or muscles?

_____ .

WHEN and under what circumstances are these sensations felt?

_____ .

Are there symptoms in OTHER AREAS that occur with your pain?

_____ .

MODALITIES

What things make the pain or other symptoms (specify) WORSE or BETTER in terms of the following categories?

TIME: (Day, night, weekly, recurring at a specific time, etc.)

_____ .

TEMPERATURE: (Hot, cold, warm room, etc.)

_____ .

WEATHER: (Damp, rainy, clear, stormy, foggy, etc.)

_____ .

POSITION: (Lying, lying on one side or the other, sitting, standing, etc.)

_____ .

MOTION: (Exercise, stretching, stooping, rest, rising up, etc.)

_____ .

BODILY ACTIVITIES: (Sleep, eating, urinating, coughing, etc.)

_____ .

SENSORY INPUT: (Touch, pressure, light, noise, smell)

_____ .

PSYCHOLOGICAL: (When studying, from anxiety, anger, with stress)

_____ .

12. CONSTITUTIONAL PRESCRIBING

TOTALITY OF SYMPTOMS

A constitutional prescription is one that includes the whole person. It seeks a remedy that will match the most central qualities of the individual as a physical, emotional, and spiritual whole. In order to match a remedy to the person we must first perceive what has been termed the *Totality of Characteristic Symptoms*. "Characteristic symptoms" means symptoms that differentiate one person from another and one remedy from another. They bear a person's stamp of individuality, and cannot be explained solely on the basis of a vague disease category or generic diagnosis. "Totality" does not imply *quantity* of symptoms, but the *quality* of each symptom in forming a cohesive idea of the remedy needed. Focusing on different aspects of this totality provides a certain flexibility in adapting to the needs of the sick person. It also provides the basis for various "schools" of homeopathy, which accent a part of the totality, like different aspects of the multifaceted gem of homeopathy (see the Prescribing Styles diagram on page 54). Below we briefly discuss the elements and categories that make up this totality of symptoms, and their relative importance.

HIERARCHY OF SYMPTOMS

A standardized way of classifying symptoms was developed by Dr. J. T. Kent, which provides a kind of three-tiered hierarchy of symptoms.

- *General Symptoms* are classified as mental (emotional and intellectual) and physical symptoms that relate to the person as a whole, symptoms for which we generally use the word "I" (I am angry; I am cold).

- *Particular Symptoms* are symptoms and modalities that arise from a local organ, tissue, or process. They are important for treating the involved area and for finding a constitutional remedy, but should not be mistaken for general symptoms. With these symptoms we often speak of the part (My stomach hurts; My feet are cold).

- *Common Symptoms* are symptoms commonly present in illness of a certain type, and being generic, are of limited use in the final choice of remedy. However, the disease category of these common symptoms may quickly lead to a small group of potential remedies that are known to be effective for that particular condition.

TOTALITY OF SYMPTOMS

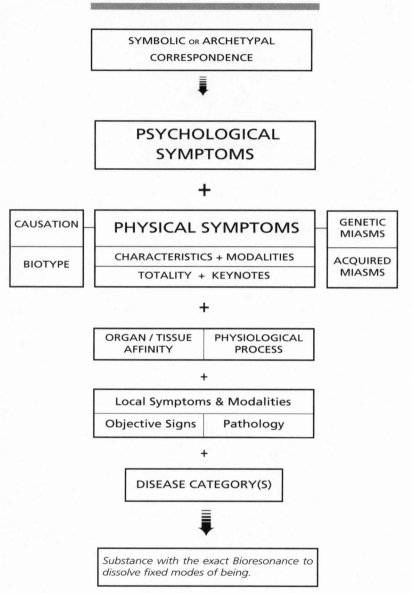

The following pages examine the different components of the total symptom picture shown in the diagram above.

1. ARCHETYPE

Archetype is the central essence or image of the patient, and of the remedy, the *pattern of meaning* that corresponds to both a natural substance and a pattern of function and structure in an individual. To directly perceive this archetype requires a deep knowledge and grasp of the essence of the remedies in the materia medica, combined with an ability to clearly perceive the person, without distortion.

2. PSYCHOLOGICAL SYMPTOMS

If a remedy matches the mental characteristics strongly, we can expect a general improvement, not just on the emotional level but in many physical symptoms, as well as in the overall health of the person. Since literally all mental and emotional processes are considered *symptoms*, the lists below are merely suggestive of the broad categories of psychological symptoms that are relevant to homeopathy.

EMOTIONAL CHARACTERISTICS

Fear • Depression • Aggression • Will (motivation and drive) • Self-esteem • Relationships (seeking company, needing to be alone) • Values (goals, purpose, ideology, etc.) • Emotional Style (open or reserved).

INTELLECTUAL CHARACTERISTICS

Intellect • Memory • Comprehension • Specific recurring thoughts or types of thoughts • Dreams (repeated or frequent dreams or images) • Perceptions (illusions, delusions) • Speed of thought or actions • Restlessness or calmness.

3. PHYSICAL GENERALS / METABOLIC SYMPTOMS

"General" or metabolic symptoms reflect the complex mix of hormonal, immunological, nutritional, hereditary, and biological factors that define a person's constitutional type. They belong to the "whole person" and thus assume a high priority in finding the remedy that matches the total individual. These symptoms include: Body temperature, Body fluids, Modalities, Desires and Aversions, Sleep, Menses, and Sexual function.

I. BODY TEMPERATURE

Temperature includes whether one is hot or chilly in general, aversion to hot or cold weather, warmth or chilliness of any part of the body (e.g. the feet), or if one part is warm and another cold simultaneously.

II. GENERAL MODALITIES

Like metabolic symptoms, general modalities affect the whole person rather than just one symptom or area. If a *local modality* shows up in several locations in the body, it can be considered a general modality.

III. DESIRES AND AVERSIONS

Desires and aversions reflect both our habits and metabolism, including:
— Abnormal craving or aversion to a specific food or beverage.
— Craving or aversion for a particular taste: salty, sweet, sour, etc.
— Thirst for cold, hot, juices, and how much one consumes at a time.
— Aggravations from specific foods or tastes, affecting the whole person.

IV. SLEEP

Sleep reflects the state of our nervous system, biochemistry, organ function, and psychology. Sleep symptoms include:
• The effects of sleep: Amelioration from sleep is normal and not of great importance. Aggravation after sleep is generally abnormal.
• Sleep disturbances: Trouble getting to sleep or staying asleep, restless or unrefreshed sleep, sleepiness, awakening at a certain time of night, etc.
• Time of day or type of sleep that affects one strongly (first sleep, nap).
• Sleeping position when first going to sleep (on the stomach, side, etc.).

V. MENSES

• Menstrual function reflects the total nutritional, neurological, and hormonal balance of the individual. The regularity, timing, duration, and flow of menses are all considered as general / metabolic symptoms.
• Also any symptom that occurs at the time of menses, or because of menses is given this same status. Symptoms of menopause, of pregnancy, and related to childbirth are similarly important.

VI. SEX

Sexual symptoms that influence the choice of constitutional remedy include the following:
— Sexual function, capabilities, impotency, infertility, etc.
— Sex drive, interest, especially if it has changed suddenly or since ill.
— Sexual activity: excess masturbation, celibacy, sexual excess.
— Aggravation or ameliorations from the sexual act.

VII. BODY FLUIDS

The fluid balance in the body and bodily secretions are highly individual and clearly reflect the state of overall health. These include:
• Perspiration: areas which perspire excessively, ease of perspiration, lack of perspiration, specific odor of the body, suppression of perspiration.
• Discharges: abnormal amounts, odors or types of discharges in general, type of mucus, excess or deficient amounts of salivation, etc.
• All these symptoms are metabolic. If they are altered due to some local disease, infection, or inflammation, they cease to be general indicators and become expressions of a local problem.

4. CAUSATION

Causative prescribing is not concerned with *speculation* or *theories* about the mechanisms of disease, but with factors that are known to have had a clear and definite impact on the health of an individual. Many of these predisposing and precipitating causes of disease are outlined in Topic 7. They might include damp climate or environment, years of physical or mental overwork, poor recovery from a variety of illnesses, or *never being well since* a fall, injury, car accident, puberty, menopause, childbirth, or after a flu or viral infection. Causes such as these, when clear and definite, are of the highest value in prescribing and are at the very core of the image of disease.

5. BIOTYPE

The most well-known remedies are related to specific physical types, such as people who are thin, heavy, flabby, with light or dark complexion or hair coloring, muscular tendency, and so on. Such typology also exists in Indian Ayurveda, Traditional Chinese Medicine, and even in the European tradition of medicine, until these ideas became unpopular early in this century. The universality of these concepts is striking.

Metabolism and structure reflect the state of the endocrine glands, one's genetic stock, and other central, constitutional factors. Metabolic and structural typology is used intensively in French homeopathy, and much less so in America. When prescribing for psychological symptoms, the biotype need not correspond, though it often does.

6. GENETIC MIASMS

As discussed, miasms are patterns of disease tendency and susceptibility. In homeopathy there are several main patterns that interact to produce most of what we know today as chronic or degenerative disease. Remedies affect one or another of these miasms, more or less deeply. Advanced homeopathic prescribing is largely concerned with the eradication of these patterns gradually over time. Prescribing on this level is also the ultimate form of prevention if initiated in early childhood.

7. ACQUIRED MIASMS

Remedies may be prescribed on the basis of particular toxic factors which leave an "imprint" or pattern in the body, and which must be neutralized or eradicated in order for the person to improve. These factors include medical and non-medical drugs, tobacco, vaccines, viral or bacterial infections that were suppressed, chemical or environmental pollutants, and specific allergens. Prescribing has become more difficult because of this multiplicity of toxic and microbial exposures.

8. ORGAN / TISSUE AFFINITY

The location of the illness is of primary importance for the selection of the right remedy in most schools of homeopathy. All remedies have a "tropism" — they each affect specific tissues and organs, and some direct almost all their force towards a single area. Some practitioners and schools of homeopathy use such remedies as *drainage* medicines to detoxify or regenerate specific organs.

9. PHYSIOLOGICAL PROCESS

Remedies have definite effects on biochemistry and physiology, and the correct remedy must match the type of disturbance that is present in the person. There are remedies that influence inflammation, others that affect tumors, and so on. Because this approach corresponds with certain concepts in mainstream medicine, hybrid systems of homeopathy have developed, seeking to bridge the medical gap and include physiological knowledge that was not available when homeopathy was first formulated. Physiological prescribing is the basis of prescribing in many parts of Europe, especially Germany. It is also the rationale for the development of many systems of low-potency combination remedies.

10. LOCAL SYMPTOMS

Local symptoms relate to sensations and disturbances that, along with their modalities, belong strictly to a single part or area. This is obvious in the case of a local injury, sprain, or infection. For constitutional prescribing, local symptoms might have minimal value, unless the symptoms or modalities that occur there are typical reactions of the person and are part of a larger pattern. Also, in many joint and musculoskeletal conditions, such as arthritis, the local problem is a reflection of a systemic disease. In such cases, mental, general, and local symptoms ultimately *all reflect the same pattern* in a different guise.

11. OBJECTIVE SIGNS

Signs are symptoms that can be seen, heard, or sensed in other ways and may reflect either local disease or constitutional problems. Some homeopathic signs are identical to those found in a typical physical exam, e.g. the state of the hair, skin, nails, types and areas of perspiration, etc., but assume a different significance, since they guide us to a choice of a homeopathic remedy. Observation can confirm reported symptoms and provide crucial insights into factors the person is unaware of, or unwilling to discuss. Objective signs are of crucial importance in infants and children, senility, insanity, animals, and in general psychological assessment.

Important objective signs in homeopathy include:
— Speech, voice, style of intonation, way of expressing words
— Clarity, concentration, coherence, presence, direction of gaze
— Mannerisms, posture, activities, gait, body language
— Emotions revealed in facial expression, voice, posture, eyes, etc.
— Observations that contradict the persons verbal report

12. PATHOLOGY

Each remedy is capable of producing specific types of physiological and pathological change, such as inflammation, ulceration, calculi, hemorrhage, bruising, or edema. Different remedies are appropriate for different degrees of tissue destruction, atrophy, scarring, etc. The correct remedy must match the make-up of the problem. Assessing the nature of the pathology can be a rapid shortcut to the group of clinically relevant remedies, both in physical and psychological disease. It is also important for determining the prognosis and curability of a condition.

13. DISEASE CATEGORIES

A whole class of homeopathic literature called *"Therapeutic Guides"* is based on the fact that the disease category brings us to a smaller group of remedies most commonly useful for this type of condition. The following section on Therapeutic Prescribing gives detailed information on this topic. *Specifics* are remedies that have an excellent track record because of their marked symptomatic, pathological, organ affinity and clinical relationship to a disease syndrome. These include remedies like Arnica for injury or Cantharis for bladder infections.

14. BIORESONANCE

Homeopathic remedies are energy medicines, each with a specific vibrational pattern that can augment the energetic qualities of the body and mind, while neutralizing disease-inducing energies. Various systems of holistic treatment, including muscle testing and electroacupuncture, seek to measure the compatibility of the organism with various healing substances. In capable hands, these methods can be quite effective in finding the "biocompatible" homeopathic remedy that can neutralize the body's illness and promote healing. Unfortunately, it can also be a substitute for lack of extensive and detailed knowledge of both homeopathic principles and materia medica. If a remedy is found to be energetically correct, but makes no sense homeopathically, the accuracy of the process is in question.

PRESCRIBING STYLES

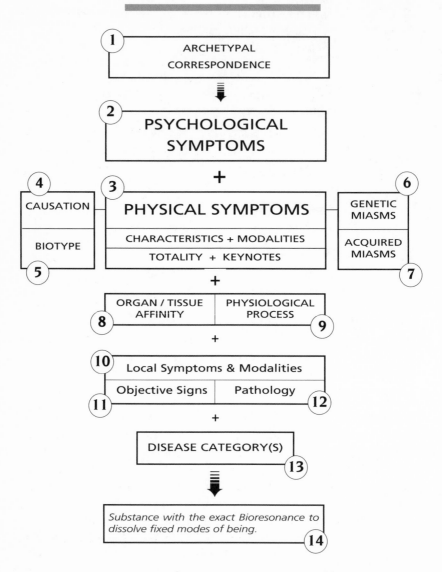

The diagram on page 48 indicates all the components of the "Totality of Symptoms." Each of these components can be used as the main, or even sole, criteria for finding the appropriate remedy. This is also the basis for various schools or systems of homeopathy that have developed over the years, each with their own specialized therapeutic focus.

13. THERAPEUTIC PRESCRIBING

Since the time of Hahnemann, homeopaths have insisted that remedies should be prescribed on the basis of the patient's unique symptoms, not the name of the disease. Though the ultimate choice of remedy depends on matching the symptoms of the patient with the symptoms of a remedy, the choice can be narrowed by choosing the group of remedies capable of curing a specific type of disease manifestation, such as arthritis. This is in fact what homeopaths have been doing for 200 years and forms the basis of *therapeutic prescribing*. Many of the famous classics of homeopathic literature are texts based on this approach.

When prescribing for a specific illnesses, a streamlined method of determining the remedy can be used, involving a four-stage process:

1. Selecting the group of remedies that have a known ability to cure the condition and the person who suffers with it.
2. From this group, selecting the remedies that match the physiological or pathological process that is going on in the body.
3. Selecting the remedies that correspond, as exactly as possible, to the unique symptoms of the individual.
4. Confirming the choice of remedy by reviewing the constitutional or general symptoms and make-up of both the patient and remedy.

If the psychological and metabolic symptoms do not correspond well, the remedy may not create a lasting or deep cure, even if it fits the musculoskeletal condition. If all symptoms correspond well, the local illness and the total health of the person should improve significantly. In the case of "smaller" remedies, the general and emotional symptoms are either not well known or not intrinsically important. Then the matching remedy will often give good results. It may be the case that, in order to accomplish deep and lasting cure, additional remedies may be needed that correspond to the psychological and biological type of the individual, i.e. constitutional remedies. Occasionally a remedy may be used that is rarely thought of or used in a particular condition, yet it is prescribed because of a few very peculiar and striking symptoms that belong to only a few remedies.

The following diagrams illustrate this four-stage process of remedy selection, giving examples of how this works in practice.

Therapeutic Prescribing

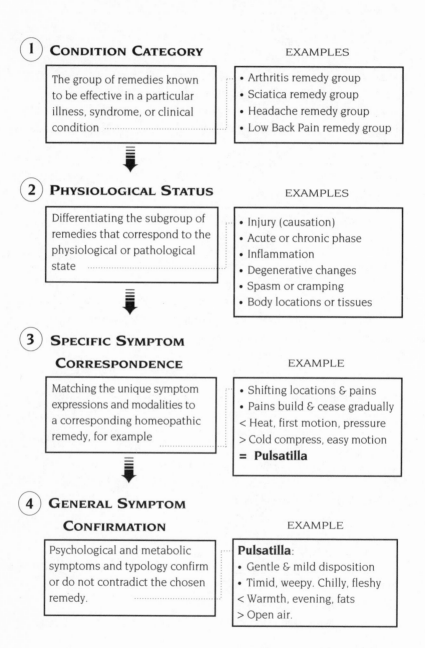

1 Condition Category   EXAMPLES

The group of remedies known to be effective in a particular illness, syndrome, or clinical condition

- Arthritis remedy group
- Sciatica remedy group
- Headache remedy group
- Low Back Pain remedy group

2 Physiological Status   EXAMPLES

Differentiating the subgroup of remedies that correspond to the physiological or pathological state

- Injury (causation)
- Acute or chronic phase
- Inflammation
- Degenerative changes
- Spasm or cramping
- Body locations or tissues

3 Specific Symptom Correspondence   EXAMPLE

Matching the unique symptom expressions and modalities to a corresponding homeopathic remedy, for example

- Shifting locations & pains
- Pains build & cease gradually
- < Heat, first motion, pressure
- > Cold compress, easy motion
- **= Pulsatilla**

4 General Symptom Confirmation   EXAMPLE

Psychological and metabolic symptoms and typology confirm or do not contradict the chosen remedy.

Pulsatilla:
- Gentle & mild disposition
- Timid, weepy. Chilly, fleshy
- < Warmth, evening, fats
- > Open air.

THERAPEUTIC EXAMPLES

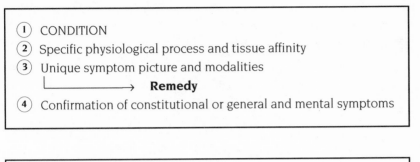

(1) CONDITION
(2) Specific physiological process and tissue affinity
(3) Unique symptom picture and modalities
└─────────→ **Remedy**
(4) Confirmation of constitutional or general and mental symptoms

---

(1) ARTHRITIS
(2) Acute inflammation with swollen, red, hot joints
(3) Stitching pain < Slightest movement > Rest, pressure, local heat
└─────────→ **Bryonia**
(4) Irritability, business worries < Cold weather > Damp and overcast

---

(1) ARTHRITIS
(2) Chronic inflammation of muscles, tendons, fibrous tissue
(3) Soreness & shooting pains < Damp, cold, night > Warmth, dry
└─────────→ **Phytolacca**
(4) Exhausted, indifferent, glandular enlargement and inflammation

---

(1) ARTHRITIS
(2) Degenerative phase; shortening of tendons, contraction of joints
(3) Drawing, burning pains < Dry weather, evenings > Damp, warm
└─────────→ **Causticum**
(4) Chronic grief. Sympathetic; sensitive to injustice.
Rebels against authority. Protects the family.

Above are typical examples of how a homeopathic medicine is chosen using a four-phase approach to remedy selection for specific conditions.

14 · POTENCY SELECTION

POTENCY

Homeopathic medicines come in standard strengths, limiting our selection to the 6, 12, 30, 200, 1M (one thousand), 10M, 50M, or CM (hundred thousand) potencies. Less often, full strength (1x or tincture), 3x or 3c are used. French manufacturers use 5c, 7c, 9c, and 15c. The selection of a particular potency is somewhat controversial, since there are numerous views, styles, and systems of prescribing. Ultimately all systems produce excellent results in the hands of a talented prescriber who understands both people and remedies. In general though, there are reliable and valuable guidelines:

- The potency directs or "aims" the remedy towards a particular biological level, with lower potencies directed towards the physical level while higher potencies are directed towards an ever subtler hierarchy of processes, energies, and biological intelligence.
- Illness exists on a particular energy level or plane within the body. The correct potency must correspond to this vibrational frequency or level to have its maximum effect in neutralizing the disturbance.
- In the course of treatment, a full range of potencies may be required, since a potency can cease to have an effect and need to be changed.
- At times the correct remedy works well in any potency, while in certain cases only the exact potency has the required effect. In any case, the right potency assures that the chosen remedy exerts its optimal effect.

POTENCY AFFINITIES

- *Very low potencies* (3x or 6x) work on a gross or material level, directly affecting the level of cells and biochemistry.
- *Low potencies* (12x, 6c, 12c) relate to specific tissues and organs.
- *Medium potencies* (30c) affect the level of *organ systems*, those complex organizations of functionally related organs and tissues such as the digestive, respiratory, or musculoskeletal systems.
- *High potencies* (200c-1M) affect the overall metabolic and control systems, including the hormonal, nervous, and immune systems.
- *Very high potencies* (10M, 50M, CM) affect the deepest levels of biology and psychology, including genetic predispositions and disease tendencies, mental complexes, and even the spiritual direction of one's life.

POTENCY GUIDELINES

LOW POTENCY

- Low potencies tend to work for shorter periods of time and act more superficially; high potencies generally act deeper and longer.
- If one is a beginner, student, or unsure of how to proceed, *don't use higher than the 30th potency*. It will still work quite well!
- When there are *few characteristic symptoms* of any one remedy on which to prescribe, use low to medium potency.
- When conditions have advanced to the point of *physical or structural changes*, lower potencies should be used.
- In such cases of *pathological change*, one can start low and possibly go gradually higher in potency over time (several months).
- Low potencies should be used in *weakened individuals* with low vitality.
- Low potency is appropriate to the *aged, small5 infants*, and *weak children*.
- Where the *response is sluggish* and there is an inability to react strongly or change quickly, low potencies are less demanding on the vitality.
- Use them in relatively "dense" or materially oriented individuals, not particularly sensitive on an intellectual, emotional, or spiritual level.
- Use low potencies where there are many *obstacles to cure*, including the long use of medical drugs, the Pill, cortisone, suppressive creams, etc.
- Where there is mental retardation, or in deaf or dumb individuals, low potencies are more commonly indicated.
- Where the *symptoms are strictly local* and when the desired effect is on a specific organ or tissue (organotherapy), use low potencies.

MEDIUM POTENCY

- The 30c or 200c is an excellent starting point for experienced practitioners. Later, one can go up or down in the scale of potencies, as needed, when an additional dose of the same remedy is required.
- When two or three remedies seem equally applicable and appropriate, a medium potency should be used for the most indicated remedy.
- In acute episodes or illnesses that are really a flare-up of a chronic disease pattern, a medium potency is recommended.
- If mainly local symptoms indicate the remedy, but there are also other indications on a general constitutional level, use a medium potency.

HIGH POTENCY

- Higher potencies are particularly effective for influencing the individual's *emotional and psychological profile* and deeper personality structure.
- Where the symptoms are clearly defined and there are many *characteristic symptoms of a single remedy*, a higher potency is well indicated.
- People who have a *strong vitality* usually respond well to high potencies.

- Where illness is *functional rather than pathological*, without serious physical disease, high potencies will be well-tolerated.
- People who are *sensitive*, spiritual, intellectual types, or people who tend to "live in their heads" generally do better on higher potencies.
- In *acute cases*, high potencies may work more quickly and effectively.
- High potencies are more *subject to antidoting* from bad diet, coffee, mint, other medicines, etc., during the initial stages after taking a remedy.
- People who have been on *many drugs* or have taken many low-potency homeopathics may require remedies in high potency.
- High potencies are usually contraindicated in *advanced pathological conditions*, where vitality is very low, in feeble children, or in advanced age.
- Both higher potencies and repeated low potencies can change the basic weakness and susceptibilities of an individual. Higher potencies start at a subtle level and work from "above down" or from the subtle to the gross physical. Low potencies gradually change the cellular basis, which ultimately has an impact on the deepest levels.

CHANGE OF POTENCY

- If a remedy seems perfect but nothing happens, try a different potency!
- A change of potency is recommended before changing remedies.
- A specific potency, whether high or low, may work for a certain time or to a certain degree, and then seem to no longer have any effect.
- If the remedy ceases to be effective when used in its original strength, the higher potency may be now be needed.
- In chronic illness, one can start low (30c) and go gradually higher over time, though Hahnemann often worked from high towards low!
- In pathological conditions, do not rush this process or ascend too quickly, but rather proceed over months or years. Thus in these cases, it is best to start relatively low, so one can go up over time.
- When a high potency fails to work at all, try using a low potency of the same remedy.

OTHER PRESCRIBING STYLES

Each of the methods below has been said by its proponents to give better, deeper reactions with less chance of a strong healing crisis:

- Five doses of the same remedy and potency 12 hours apart.
- Two doses of different potencies (e.g. 200c and 1M) given 24 or 48 hours apart from each other.
- Three sequential potencies (6, 30c, 200c or 30c, 200c, 1M etc.) given on three successive days (the method of Kent and Tyler).
- The LM system, in which remedies are diluted on the basis of 1 to 50,000, has strong adherents in both America and India.

15. TAKING THE REMEDY

THE DOSAGE

SUGAR

A dose is usually three or four sugar pills (depending on size of pellets), dissolved in the mouth 30 minutes away from foods, tastes, or flavorings that might interfere with subtle remedy action. Since these are energy medicines rather than chemical drugs the number of pellets is not crucial; the reason for administering several pellets is to make sure that one has received a pellet that has been saturated with the remedy.

WATER

Liquid remedies are often given in doses of 10 drops, though labels should be followed. Also, a few pellets or drops stirred in a glass of water will energize its entire contents, and this can be used in teaspoonful doses for frequent repetitions. Spring water should be used and the glass covered and kept out of the light. A fresh solution should be made after a day or two. Afterwards, the glass must be boiled or heated at high temperature (a dishwasher works well) to remove all traces of the medicine's presence, which may keep the glass "charged up."

THE SINGLE DOSE

- Generally one remedy is used at a time
- If more than one remedy seems indicated, these can be alternated.
- If alternating remedies are used, they should be taken some hours apart from each other, noting the effects of each.

ADMINISTRATION

Remedies work via the nervous system and subtle energy of the body, rather than relying on absorption into the blood stream for their action. Thus any area *rich in sensitive nerves* is an appropriate route of administration: the tongue, skin, nose, eye, rectum, etc.

MOUTH

- Pellets should be placed in the clean mouth, free of all tastes or odors of foods, beverages, etc. These sugar pellets are allowed to dissolve *on or under the tongue*, rather that swallowing or chewing.
- Most texts advise putting homeopathics medicines *under* the tongue to avoid contact with food or other substances.

- Liquid remedies or water with remedies dissolved in it should be held in the mouth. They can be also be rubbed on the lips of a small child.

NOSE

The method which gives the quickest effect and which is suitable to *highly allergic and sensitive individuals* is to simply sniff an open bottle of the remedy. This is one dose. Because of its subtle nature, this method is not always reliable.

TIME OF ADMINISTRATION

- The best time to give a remedy is before *and not during* its particular time of worsening or aggravation (time of day, season, during menses, etc.). Times of aggravation are found in most materia medica.
- Do not give a chronic, deep-acting remedy during an acute illness or crisis. Wait until the crisis is over, as the body's main priority and focus at that point is resolving the acute condition.

FREQUENCY OF DOSE

- Frequency of dose depends on the severity of the condition, the potency, and the duration and depth of the remedy's action.
- Some remedies are short acting and require frequent repetition, while others rarely need it even in acute illness.
- Information about the duration and relative depth of action of remedies is usually given in materia medica, including the one in this book.

ACUTE CONDITIONS

- In acute conditions, remedies can be given frequently, as the body "uses up" the remedy quickly and requires another dose.
- *When symptoms are very intense*: In the initial phases give a dose every 15 minutes for the first hour or longer. With improvement, reduce to hourly doses. In severe injury continue this for the first day or even two. Reduce to every two hours with further improvement. After several days reduce the repetition to three times daily. *The number of pellets is always the same.*
- *For moderate or mild symptoms*: Remedies can be taken anywhere from every two hours (6 times daily) to three times daily, depending on the intensity and severity of symptoms. Reduce gradually with improvement.

CHRONIC CONDITIONS

- Certain remedies for chronic illness which are given in medium or low potency can be taken daily or weekly on a regular basis.
- Other remedies, as indicated in the Materia Medica section, require only infrequent doses. In this case the remedy is repeated according to the degree of reaction or improvement (see Topic 16).

REPETITION OF THE DOSE

- When people are sensitive and the remedy is clear, a single dose can be used (depending on the relative depth of action of the remedy).
- When many allopathic drugs are being used, frequent repetitions of the homeopathic remedy may be required to get a positive response.
- In *acute conditions* the remedy is often repeated on a regular basis until improvement is definitely noted. Then the remedy is given less often or is not repeated until symptoms indicate the need.
- When using higher potencies in *chronic conditions*, the remedy does not have to be repeated until the first dose has finished working, which may be several weeks or even months.
- It requires careful observation to see if there is improvement (even subtlely) or a temporary worsening i.e. healing crisis.
- When using lower potencies in chronic disease (below 30c), remedies can be repeated daily, once or twice for several weeks or more, depending on how long improvement seems to last.
- In very long-term conditions, it may take remedies some time to begin showing positive effects — up to four weeks in some cases.

DURATION OF TREATMENT

- In general, remedies only need be given *until the body reacts*.
- Once a remedy has initiated a healing response, this should be allowed to run its course. Sometimes one course of treatment will initiate healing processes that require months or years for completion. Meanwhile both the general health and disease condition improve incrementally.
- *Acute conditions* are self-limiting, and remedies can greatly accelerate the healing process.
- The time needed for the treatment of *chronic conditions* corresponds to their depth, severity, and duration.
- A sciatica of several months standing may only require a few weeks of treatment, whereas advanced arthritis requires many months or even years of systematic care.
- Remedies can be continued for up to a month in low potency.
- If longer treatment is required, stop or substitute remedies for one week and then resume, continuing in this way to administer the remedy for three weeks out of four.
- Ultimately the ill person, as expressed in their symptom picture, should be the guide to when, or how often a remedy is needed.

CARE OF HOMEOPATHIC REMEDIES

Remedies are sensitive and can be antidoted in various ways:
- ODORS: Opening a remedy in the presence of strong perfumes, moth balls, incense, or aromatic oils may ruin the whole bottle.
- TIME: In spite of labels that are required by law to state an expiry date, remedies may last for a century or more — unless antidoted by any of the factors listed here.
- CAMPHOR: Camphor has a general antidotal effect on many remedies and should be kept far away from homeopathic remedies. It is found in various liniments, "tiger balm," and camphorated ointments.
- LIGHT: Light is an enemy of homeopathic substances, as its strong photon activity will disrupt the energy pattern of the remedy. Prolonged exposure to bright sunlight or strong fluorescent lights can completely "zap" remedies, leaving them less effective or useless.
- HEAT: Strong heat, above 110°F, can neutralize remedies. If a remedy is left in a glove compartment in summer heat, it is likely damaged.
- PACKAGING MATERIALS: Because of the above considerations, remedies must be in containers that are impervious to light and made of a non-porous substance. Certain specialized plastics are acceptable, though glass is the traditional medium, either of a dark color, or with a label that excludes all light. Cheap plastic will off-gas toxins into the remedy and is porous enough to allow contamination.
- MAGNETIC FIELDS: Electrical and magnetic fields can neutralize remedies. This includes metal detectors and close proximity to computers, television screens, clock radios, and other electrical devices.
- X-RAY: Exposure to X-ray will partially or completely ruin remedies.
- STORAGE: Keep remedies in a dark place at room temperature or in their own filing card box. Do not store in refrigerators, spice cabinets, with herbs, near chemicals and cleansers, or near any other strong-smelling substances. This precludes storage in most medicine cabinets.
- SPECIFIC ANTIDOTES: Each remedy has special relationships, both positive and negative, with other remedies. A list of complementary and antidotal remedies is found in the Appendix.
- LIFESTYLE: All the negative modalities or aggravations of a homeopathic medicine are things that a person taking that remedy should avoid, such as damp, cold, certain positions, etc. There are also specific food aggravations for each remedy which can be found in larger materia medica. It is useful to avoid foods that are antidotal or aggravate your remedy-type.

CARE OF HOMEOPATHIC PATIENTS

The positive effects of a remedy on the body and mind can be partially or even completely interrupted or antidoted by things that interfere with the healing trends of the organism:

- DRUGS: Excess alcohol consumption, marijuana, tobacco, cocaine, and other toxic drugs can easily have these antidotal effects.
- COFFEE: Traditionally coffee is considered a common antidote to homeopathic remedies. This is not always the case, but how can one know until after the fact? Generally it is advisable to reduce or eliminate coffee while undergoing homeopathic treatment, unless there is so much psychological resistance that it outweighs the potential benefit.
- MINT is also considered a general antidote to remedy action. Though one episode of mint tea or toothpaste will not destroy the effect of a deep remedy, its regular use should be suspended during treatment.
- TRAUMA: A serious injury or accident may disrupt the action of a remedy. This is logical, as the priority of the body shifts to taking care of business around the trauma one has received.
- EMOTIONS: Similarly, a severe emotional shock such as death, a personal loss, or an extreme fright can disrupt and halt the action of remedies. Prolonged periods of extreme stress can also have this effect.
- MEDICAL DRUGS: Unfortunately, some medical drugs can make remedies less effective or not work at all. This is logical, since these two types of medicine are often working in opposite directions. A homeopathic remedy is supporting natural processes and biological intelligence, while a conventional medical drug is suppressing both. Many times though, remedies will still be effective, and since they do not negatively affect medical drugs, they can be used simultaneously.
- SURGERY: Major surgery, or even dental work, can be a significant enough shock or trauma to divert the body from its healing work.
- NATURAL THERAPIES: Many practitioners find acupuncture, nutritional supplements, spinal manipulation, etc., to be highly compatible and synergistic with homeopathy. Others feel that homeopathics should be used alone. In any case, too many therapies do make it difficult to know which treatment is having the most significant effect.
- When a remedy has been antidoted, it often just means that it must be repeated. Be patient however, and really observe whether the remedy is no longer having an effect, rather than assuming it is so.
- NOTE that if the homeopathic remedy is *precisely for* the mental stress, emotional trauma, drug or alcohol abuse, etc., there will be no interference with from that factor. On the contrary, the condition will be helped.

16. THE HEALING PROCESS

THE JOURNEY TO HEALTH

We are accustomed to a suppressive form of health care, where results are relatively quick, yet superficial. This approach has little real relationship to the normal biological needs or intentions of the body. Thus we are unfamiliar with the *process of healing*, which follows very specific patterns and pathways and which can be recognized and assisted. This section describes some of the most important themes and concepts for understanding what happens after a remedy is given.

BIOLOGICAL TIME

Everywhere in nature we see the pervasive influence of biological time. Growth, decay, and healing all require their own unique period, from the regeneration of organs to the cleansing and detoxification of tissue. Natural medicine in general and homeopathy in particular can initiate and accelerate healing and reactivate what was stuck or unavailable. Yet it is still bound to natural processes, which can be remarkably fast and efficient, but do involve time, whether in minutes or years.

HEALING CRISIS

As described earlier, some symptom patterns are expressions of the healing process, which may entail uncomfortable symptoms. Both lay people and practitioners are quite familiar with the old adage that "you have to get worse before you get better." Though this may often be the case, it obviously does not mean that worse is *always* better, or that feeling worse after taking a natural remedy is necessarily good! In fact there are very specific signs and points of differentiation to distinguish between just getting worse (a disease crisis), and an actual healing crisis, which we will examine in the next few pages. In general, the most intense healing crisis is likely to occur in the initial stages of homeopathic therapy. Over time, the organism strengthens and develops more sensitivity and facility in navigating the healing process.

THE HEALING PROCESS

Because of the complexity and many layers of cause which exist for each person, the healing process is not a homogenous, monotone process. The process will unfold in its highly unique way, exactly according to the capabilities of the person, the healing stimulus that is applied, and the obstacles to cure.

- Diagram A on the following page shows the gradual process of healing, the hills and valleys in this graph mirroring the internal struggle and revolution of health that is taking place in the individual.
- *Healing phases* occur in which there is a regular and marked improvement in the condition and in the individual.
- *Plateau phases* occur when, for a period of time, the body maintains an improved state, but goes no further. This does not necessarily mean that more heroic, stronger methods are needed to promote healing.
- Plateaus are times of consolidation, rest, and gathering of resources, enabling the organism to mount further incursions into health.

DECREASE IN SYMPTOMS

As we know, there are different types and levels of symptoms, which have different values and meanings relative to our total health. With healing and cure we expect symptoms to improve, but the order in which this happens is crucial.

In Diagram B, there are three symptom categories shown by three lines. In a successful healing process, the vitality and energy should gradually improve. Symptoms related to the deepest organs, structures, and mechanisms should steadily decrease. More superficial, local symptoms may fluctuate, at times worsening, but eventually subsiding.

HERING'S GUIDELINES TO CURE

- The body does not cure in a haphazard or meaningless fashion.
- At any point in time the body has a very definite and defined set of biochemical, biological, and energetic resources at its command. It thus demonstrates extreme selectivity and purpose in its healing priorities.
- Simply, it will make every effort to cure the sickest part first, and then move on to the next most important area, and so on.
- The healing process has been observed and studied since remotest antiquity by those in the tradition of natural healing, including Hippocrates, Paracelsus, and Avicenna. In homeopathy, Dr. Constantine Hering reaffirmed and restated the facts about how the organism undertakes curing itself in his famous "Laws of Cure" as outlined below.
- Biological healing is governed by the following priorities:

  1. From more important, essential organs to less important areas

  2. From the center to the periphery, or from within outwards

  3. From above downwards

  4. In reverse chronological order of the onset of the problem

- Thus, as current symptoms improve, *old, previously unresolved symptoms often arise*, like peeling the layers of an onion.

THE HEALING PROCESS

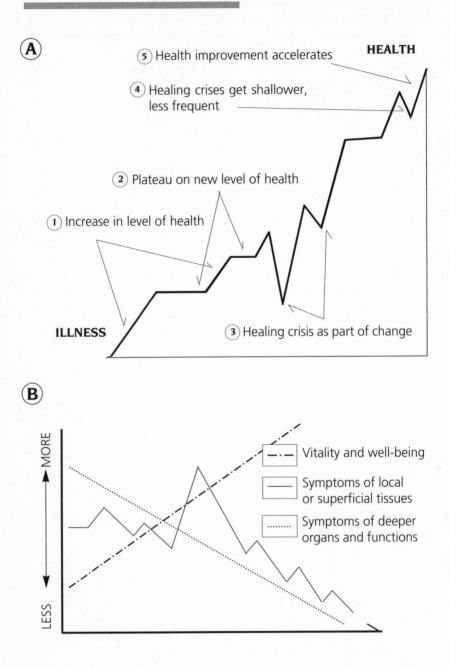

THE HIERARCHY OF ORGANS

The biological intelligence of the body has a clear priority in protecting the health of tissues that are the most valuable for survival. These tissues are often made of cells that cannot be replaced and do not regenerate (nervous system or heart) and have a high "maintenance cost," requiring large amounts of oxygen and nutrients. Other tissues are relatively less valuable to the body, requiring little nutrition (fat cells), while some are dispensable because of being highly regenerative and able to handle significant damage without severely compromising the body as a whole (digestive linings, skin). Some tissues are absolutely essential to life each moment and must be supported at all costs. Others are lower on the scale of priorities and their maintenance is less important. A partial list of the hierarchy of organs is shown below in decreasing order of importance:

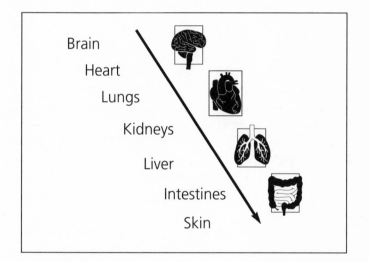

Brain
Heart
Lungs
Kidneys
Liver
Intestines
Skin

DEPTH OF PATHOLOGY

In addition to the body's hierarchy, the other factor determining the priority of an illness is the nature of the condition and how advanced the particular disease process is. A superficial tissue (skin) can have a very advanced, life-threatening disease (cancer). Or a very vital organ (heart) can have a superficial condition (palpitations). It is the interplay of the depth of tissue and degree of pathology that makes a particular problem the true "chief complaint."

This is where the organism — body and mind — focuses its considerable force in order to change and resolve the situation.

THE REMEDY RESPONSE

The healing process evolves over time and according to biological laws, but how do we know if a remedy is having a truly curative effect? Next to finding the right remedy in the first place, this is the single most vital question facing a homeopathic prescriber.

- In *constitutional prescribing*, where one dose of a remedy may be left to work for weeks and months, deciding if a remedy is working correctly — or working at all — can be complex.
- In *therapeutic prescribing* and when high potencies are not being used, the action of the remedy may be apparent sooner, and its relative effectiveness more obvious.
- In any healing process, the yardstick of change is Hering's Guidelines of Cure, which helps determine if the direction of cure is progressing positively, negatively, or just reacting partially.

LAYERS OF DISEASE

In an ideal situation, where the constitution is strong and uncomplicated, one remedy will work on all aspects of the illness, mental and physical symptoms, and the underlying weaknesses. If the remedy chosen is fairly good, but not the *perfect* match for the symptom picture, only some of the symptoms will be helped. If a follow-up remedy is needed, one that is complementary to the first remedy is often indicated (see Appendix for remedy relationships). But in many cases disease becomes very complex and intertwined with the vital force. As different layers of the person's illness are stripped away, different remedies are required for progress. By the same token, *therapeutic* prescriptions may require *constitutional* follow-up.

TYPES OF RESPONSE

- Basically only four things can occur after taking a remedy:
  1. There is no change
  2. This is improvement
  3. There is worsening
  4. There is change or something new happening.
- These changes can relate to the general sense of well-being, energy, and health, or only to specific symptoms, locations, or problems.
- The accompanying table shows some of the most common types of remedy reactions, particularly if a constitutional remedy is given.
- Homeopathic treatment is not a one-shot, suppressive treatment, but requires careful guidance of the healing process over time.
- Remedy responses and healing reactions can be confusing. For serious and advanced conditions, expert professional consultation is necessary.

No Effect

- Wrong remedy.
- Wrong potency.
- Remedy was antidoted.
- Patient is a slow reactor.
- Remedy is a slow-acting one.
- Patient has very low vitality.
- Person does not admit change.
- There is deep miasmatic block.

Interpretation

- Consider the 2nd or 3rd choice remedies.
- Try a higher or lower potency.
- Check interfering factors, drugs, lifestyle.
- Give high potency, or frequent low dose.
- Wait at least a month after high potency.
- Potency was too high, remedy too deep.
- Reassess symptom responses.
- Use deeper remedy, nosode, higher dose.

Better

- Improvement on all levels.
- Short improvement only.
- Briefly worse, then improves.
- Long aggravation, slowly better.
- Improvement finally ceases.
- Improvement, then a little worse, but better than at first.

Interpretation

- Right remedy, potency, no pathology.
- Remedy or potency too superficial, remedy antidoted, or advanced disease.
- Short healing crisis. Very good.
- Long healing crisis. condition was advanced. Use remedies carefully.
- If symptoms the same, repeat remedy.
- Remedy is working, but the person is impatient.

Worse

- Improves quickly, then much worse or just gets worse.
- Symptoms worse, but also stopping other drugs, coffee, etc.
- Severe aggravation, though the person seems strong and vital.

Interpretation

- Poor prognosis, pathology is very deep or vitality too low. Remedy not taking hold or might be too strong.
- Reactivation of suppressed condition or experiencing withdrawal symptoms.
- Potency too high, or low potency was repeated too often.

Change

- Improves, but some old symptoms return, temporarily.
- Improved; eventually new, more superficial symptoms remain.
- Improves, but new, worse symptoms appear, deeper than first.
- Improves, but some new symptoms that belong to remedy.
- Symptoms were vague, chaotic, now they are clear, localized.

Interpretation

- Recurrence of symptoms as part of action of first remedy, allow them to work through.
- If new symptom picture takes the forefront, prescribe new remedy for it.
- Reaction is going in the wrong direction; remedy needs to be antidoted or wait.
- A proving is occurring. Good remedy, but not perfect. Extra symptoms will subside.
- Very good indication. Prescribe for new clarified symptoms.

Condition Charts

CONDITION CHARTS

THE MUSCULOSKELETAL SYSTEM

1. JOINTS

• Our joints are complex structures designed for varying mixtures of strength and stability, combined with flexibility and mobility. They hold us in the posture we want to be and allow us to move where we wish to go.

• The synovial membrane is the smooth lining of the joint compartment, rich in nerve and blood supply, that provides lubricating synovial fluid. This synovia is often the first site of joint inflammation (synovitis).

2. LIGAMENTS

• Ligaments hold joints together, help guide their movement, and limit their range of motion, providing stability and strength. At rest, our joints often "hang by the ligaments" so that little muscle tension is needed. They are highly pain-sensitive structures.

• Capsular ligaments encircle the entire joint, while others support its sides. Ligaments can be overstretched (strains) or damaged and torn (sprains). Through overuse or repeated strains there can be gradual overstretching or weakening of joints (ligamentous laxity), making them unstable and subject to further trauma. Ligaments can become stiff and contracted with underuse or joint disease and are a common site of adhesions.

3. MUSCLE

Opposing groups of muscles perform complementary functions, acting as pulleys on the levers of bone, making all our complex movements in the world possible. Muscles can be strained or pulled, with familiar soreness and aching. They spasm when irritated, and are familiar sites of chronic tension or excess tone. Muscle inflammation (myositis) can be local or may occur across diffuse areas with the formation of painful nodules (trigger points). Muscles can also weaken and atrophy, particularly with arthritic joints whose painfulness reduces movement drastically.

4. TENDON

Muscles taper down to fibrous bands with which they attach to bones. Tendons and their linings can become painfully inflamed (tendonitis or tenosynovitis) or can be seriously damaged or torn, as is typical in chronic shoulder problems. Tendons can rupture, requiring plastic surgery.

5. CARTILAGE

Articular cartilage is the glass-like lining of the ends of bones that creates a smooth, low-friction joint surface. With very poor blood supply, injury to this cartilage heals poorly and slowly. Arthritic changes occur when this surface becomes pitted, cracked, and brittle. Other cartilage is highly elastic attaching bones to form a spongy and flexible joint. This is typical of the spine where the cartilage discs that join vertebrae are subject to wear and tear, thinning, bulging, and fragmentation.

6. BURSA

Bursa are fluid-filled sacs around joints that act as cushions or lubricating pads to allow a smooth gliding surface between tendons and bones or other tissues. The bursa around large joints (knee, shoulder, hips, elbows) can become inflamed after injury, resulting in bursitis.

7. BONE

Bone is an active tissue, forming and remodeling constantly in response to the physical stresses and structural demands put on the body. At sites of continued excess pressure or traction, bone will respond by overgrowth, creating bone spurs or osteophytes. With chronic joint inflammation or hormonal and mineral imbalance, bone will lose substance and increase in brittleness (osteoporosis).

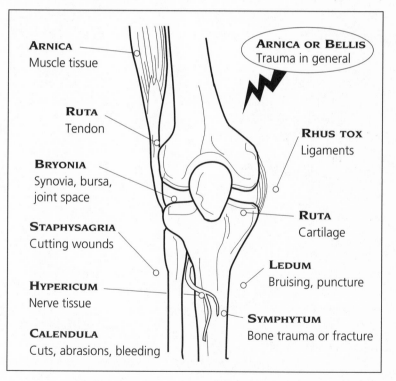

ARNICA
Muscle tissue

ARNICA OR BELLIS
Trauma in general

RUTA
Tendon

RHUS TOX
Ligaments

BRYONIA
Synovia, bursa, joint space

RUTA
Cartilage

STAPHYSAGRIA
Cutting wounds

LEDUM
Bruising, puncture

HYPERICUM
Nerve tissue

SYMPHYTUM
Bone trauma or fracture

CALENDULA
Cuts, abrasions, bleeding

BASIC REMEDY / TISSUE AFFINITIES

PAIN

Pain is a biochemical, neurological, and psychological event that occurs when an impulse, stimulated by tissue changes, travels through nervous pathways and reaches the brain. Muscle, ligament, bone coverings, joint linings, and the nerve itself are all capable of inducing pain. From a medical or diagnostic point of view, the way a pain "feels" is often irrelevant; in homeopathy the subjective quality of the pain is *extremely useful* in finding the correct and appropriate curative remedy. Though in the habit of ignoring the subtleties of pain (since nobody wants to hear about it!), we need to be attentive and "listen" to painful sensations as part of the rich and *meaningful* symptom language of the body.

QUALITY OF PAIN

- SHARP: Cutting (a knife that slices), Stabbing (a knife plunging in), Piercing (a slender knife that goes deeply), Stitching (with a needle), Pricking (like a pin), Splinter-like, Stinging (like a bee sting).
- RADIATING pains radiate from the original area. Shooting (rapid and fairly far), Darting (sharper and shorter distance), Lancinating (shooting with a deeper piercing pain), or extending and staying in a remote area.
- ACHING: Dull ache (overused muscles), Soreness (slightly sharper), as if bruised (a diffuse ache), intense aching (an unrelenting toothache).
- TENDERNESS to touch is often associated with an ache, but may also be very sharp or produce other sensations.
- PRESSURE: Pressing (inward) or Drawing.(outwards). Pressing pain can be like thumb pressure, a weight, or may intensify to a Crushing pain.
- SHARP & PRESSURE combinations produce Digging (small and penetrating), Boring (like a drill), Twisting (like a corkscrew), Pinching (try it if not sure!), Gnawing (as on a bone), Tearing (pulling and sharp).
- ANALOGOUS: Pains may be described according to familiar sensations such as "as if sprained," "as if broken," "as if dislocated," Lame (causing an inability to function or move), Paralytic (even more so).
- CIRCULATORY: Pulsating, Throbbing, Bursting, Hammering (in or out).
- SENSATION: Pain combined with strong sensations can be Burning, Icy cold needles, Tingling pain, Numbing pain, etc.
- SPASM: Tension (tight muscle), Cramping (tightening up and releasing), Spastic or Tensive pain, Contractive, Constrictive or Band-like pains.
- CONSISTENCY: The quality (or intensity) of pain may stay the same or be Changeable or Erratic. There may be several coexistent pains.

TYPES of PAIN

TIMING:
- Constant
- Recurrent
- Episodic
- Paroxysmal
- Remittent

SORE: Aching
"Bruised"
Dull ache

TENDER:
Sensitive

LOCALIZATION:
- Small spots
- Diffuse
- Spreading
- Changing

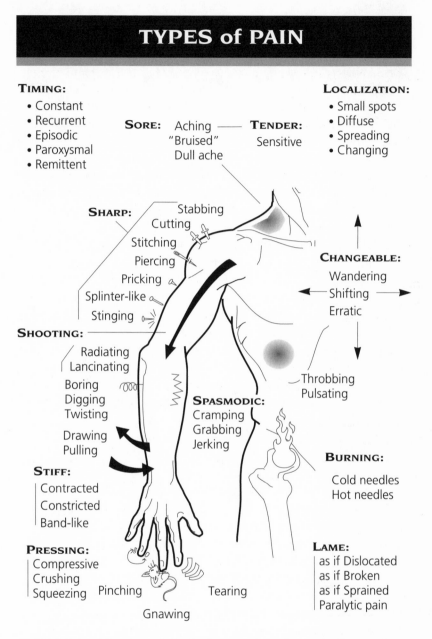

SHARP: Stabbing
Cutting
Stitching
Piercing
Pricking
Splinter-like
Stinging

CHANGEABLE:
Wandering
Shifting
Erratic

SHOOTING:
Radiating
Lancinating
Boring
Digging
Twisting

Drawing
Pulling

SPASMODIC:
Cramping
Grabbing
Jerking

Throbbing
Pulsating

STIFF:
Contracted
Constricted
Band-like

BURNING:
Cold needles
Hot needles

PRESSING:
Compressive
Crushing
Squeezing   Pinching   Tearing

Gnawing

LAME:
as if Dislocated
as if Broken
as if Sprained
Paralytic pain

NOTE: *Pain is not the only criteria for choosing a remedy*, as the many other sensations, associated symptoms, modalities (things which make the pain worse or better), causes and initiating factors are all important.

1

SENSATIONS & SIGNS

SENSATIONS

Neurologically, pain is due to a combination of heat, touch, pressure, and pain receptors in the tissues. Yet the source of the rich matrix of sensations that we experience may lie in the much subtler direction of "bioenergy," beyond brain and chemistry. In any case, in the context of the musculoskeletal system, these highly individual symptoms occur from nerve compression or irritation (sciatica or neuralgia), nerve inflammation (neuritis), or from all kinds of biochemical, inflammatory, or mechanical influences on the tissues. The most important sensations include the following:

- STIFFNESS: from muscle spasm, adhesions, swelling, bony obstruction.
- PARESTHESIAS: abnormal sensations that include crawling, formication, prickling, as if asleep, itching, tingling, or numbness (anesthesia), excess ticklishness, hyperesthesia (oversensitivity).
- ODD SENSATIONS: the part feels expanded, separated from the body, internal trembling, bubbling or boiling, as if something loose inside.
- TEMPERATURE: heat, burning, or coldness of a part, cold or hot swelling.
- MOTOR disturbances may be due to simple exhaustion, involvement of nerves, or be secondary to trauma, inflammation, or systemic disease. They include weakness, heaviness, awkwardness, lack of co-ordination, local paralysis, or on the other hand, spasm, cramps, trembling, or twitching.

SYMPTOMS AND SIGNS

Signs are symptoms that can be clearly and objectively observed. The most typical signs occurring in musculoskeletal conditions are:

- SWELLING: Swelling is commonly seen with injury and inflammation, and is associated with many remedies. Differentiating factors include color of the area (red, white, pale, waxy, bruised), temperature (hot, cold), painful or painless, degree of tenderness, location in the body, etc.
- DEFORMITY: Contraction and shortening of muscles and tendons, or tightness and adhesions of ligaments create joint deformities, reduce mobility, and are experienced as constrictive sensations.
- BONE CHANGES: Nodules, nodosities, protrusions, hard swellings.
- RESTLESSNESS may be due to nervousness and anxiety, to efforts to reduce pain or stiffness, or to a neurological condition. Desire for rest or stillness and aversion to motion are also important.
- POSTURE: Position of the spine: stooped, leaning. Position of a limb or area: arm, wrist, or knee held bent, foot turned in, etc.
- ACTIVITY: Unable to rise, limping, stretching, lying still, etc.

SENSATIONS & SYMPTOMS

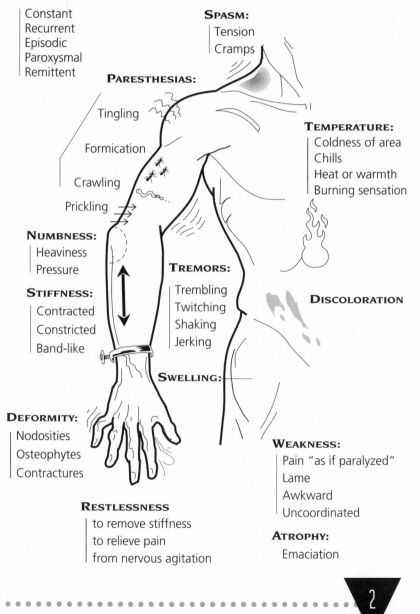

FREQUENCY OF SYMPTOM:
Constant
Recurrent
Episodic
Paroxysmal
Remittent

SPASM:
Tension
Cramps

PARESTHESIAS:
Tingling
Formication
Crawling
Prickling

TEMPERATURE:
Coldness of area
Chills
Heat or warmth
Burning sensation

NUMBNESS:
Heaviness
Pressure

STIFFNESS:
Contracted
Constricted
Band-like

TREMORS:
Trembling
Twitching
Shaking
Jerking

DISCOLORATION

DEFORMITY:
Nodosities
Osteophytes
Contractures

SWELLING:

WEAKNESS:
Pain "as if paralyzed"
Lame
Awkward
Uncoordinated

RESTLESSNESS
to remove stiffness
to relieve pain
from nervous agitation

ATROPHY:
Emaciation

2

TRAUMA

The human frame, for all its remarkable capacities is, alas, not invincible. From simple scratches to devastating and fatal injury, trauma is the most common and pervasive medical condition encountered. The complex ways in which the body deals with injury are also a vivid demonstration of the intelligent and coordinated "response-ability" of the body.

The remarkable effects of homeopathy for injury are unrivaled, as there are no analogous medical drugs that can stimulate repair and accelerate healing of damaged tissue, while reducing pain, swelling, bruising, secondary infection, and preventing the long-term residual effects of trauma. This is the power of *assisting biology*, rather than *suppressing it*.

TRAUMA can occur in any part of the body: soft tissue, hard tissue, skin, organs, etc. For our purposes the most important injuries are those that have immediate and long-term effects on the musculoskeletal system.

• Arnica is the most renowned trauma remedy, and is without equal as the primary remedy for injury of any kind whatsoever, to be followed by other more specific remedies depending on the area and type of trauma.

• Remedies for bruising, bleeding, fracture, sprains, and so on are listed in the Therapeutic Guide, with additional comments below.

• BRUISING: Arnica, Bellis, Ledum, and Sulphuric acid are the main remedies for bruising, in exactly that order of severity and chronicity.

• BLEEDING: There are dozens of remedies for hemorrhage. The main remedies for bleeding from injury include Hamamelis and Phosphorus.

• SEQUELAE are the long-term after-effects of injury. These include symptoms that never go away, health that never returns to normal, and the development of problems such as arthritis even many years later. Homeopathy is the first choice when a person has "never been well" since a specific traumatic incidence. Arnica and Hypericum are the main remedies, prescribed in high potency for several doses, for erasing the imprints of trauma within the nervous system and tissues. Rhus tox, Ruta, and Hamamelis can have similar benefits. Other symptoms that may follow injury include fear (Aconitum and Arnica), depression (Nat sulph), exhaustion (Carbo veg), and inflammation (Rhus tox, Ruta, Phytolacca).

• FRACTURE: Arnica is used first for one or two weeks, once or twice daily. Ledum can be alternated with Arnica after 24 hours to help with the internal and external bruising. Symphytum used daily in low potency or once weekly in the 200th greatly accelerates healing, as does Ruta. Hypericum should be used if there has been nerve injury.

TRAUMATIC MAN

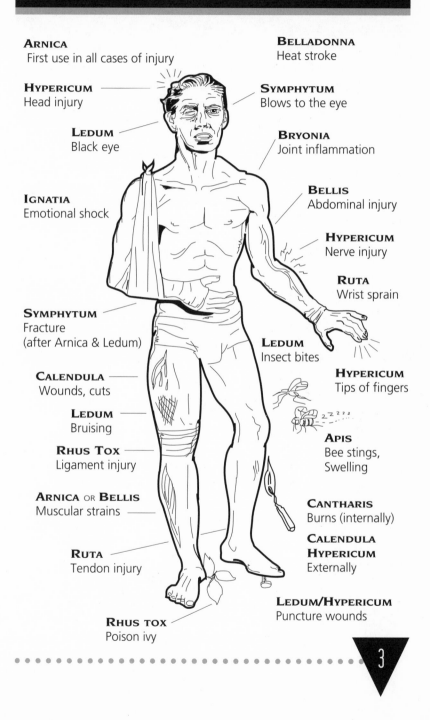

ARNICA
First use in all cases of injury

BELLADONNA
Heat stroke

HYPERICUM
Head injury

SYMPHYTUM
Blows to the eye

LEDUM
Black eye

BRYONIA
Joint inflammation

IGNATIA
Emotional shock

BELLIS
Abdominal injury

HYPERICUM
Nerve injury

RUTA
Wrist sprain

SYMPHYTUM
Fracture
(after Arnica & Ledum)

LEDUM
Insect bites

CALENDULA
Wounds, cuts

HYPERICUM
Tips of fingers

LEDUM
Bruising

RHUS TOX
Ligament injury

APIS
Bee stings,
Swelling

ARNICA OR **BELLIS**
Muscular strains

CANTHARIS
Burns (internally)

CALENDULA
HYPERICUM
Externally

RUTA
Tendon injury

LEDUM/HYPERICUM
Puncture wounds

RHUS TOX
Poison ivy

3

TRAUMA 1

Injury: Main Remedies

- 1st remedy for TRAUMA, shock. Restless, fearful.
- Muscular strains. Bruising. Before & after exercise.
- Sore bruised sensation < TOUCH, jar, motion, night.

ARNICA 7
Muscle

- Injury to NERVES or nerve-rich tissues; neuralgia.
- Blows to the spine or head, coccyx, fingers, toes.
- Pains shoot upward from injury < TOUCH, jar, cold.

HYPERICUM 32
Nerve

- Trauma to deep tissue layers; abdomen, legs, pelvis.
- SWELLING, bruising, soreness. Prolonged standing.
- Recurrent trauma; REPETITIVE STRAIN. > Rubbing.

BELLIS 11
Deep tissues

- Sprains, falls, dislocations, injury to tendon, bone.
- Muscle strains. Pain of fracture. Fever after injury.
- < Slight MOTION, touch > *immobilization*, cold, pressure.

BRYONIA 13
Joint linings

- Blows, joint sprains, muscular strains, OVERLIFTING.
- STIFFNESS. Restless. Strained voice. Tearing pains.
- < *First motion*, after rest, damp, cold > Limbering, heat.

RHUS TOX 47
Ligament

- *Injury* or *strain* to joint, tendon, cartilage, periosteum.
- Dislocation, fracture, sprains, overexertion. *Weak joints*.
- < Motion (but restless), sitting, cold. Joint deposits.

RUTA 48
Tendon - Cartilage

- FRACTURE, broken bones, poor healing, concussion.
- Injury to eye, face, shins, *periosteum*, cartilage, tendons.
- Pain in old fractures or wounds. *Pain after amputation*.

SYMPHYTUM 58
Bone

4 •

TRAUMA 2

Additional Useful Remedies

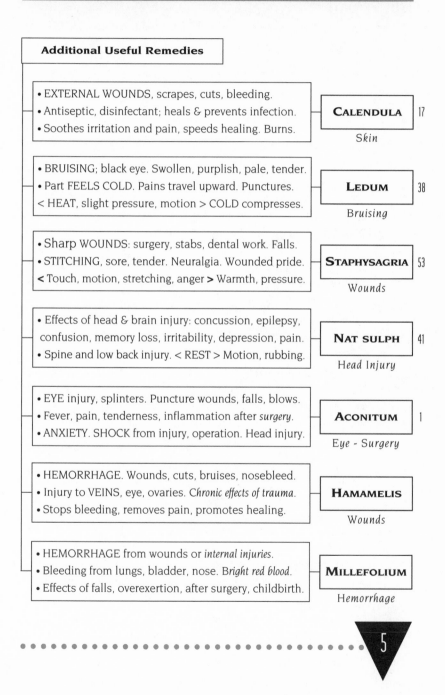

- EXTERNAL WOUNDS, scrapes, cuts, bleeding.
- Antiseptic, disinfectant; heals & prevents infection.
- Soothes irritation and pain, speeds healing. Burns.

CALENDULA 17
Skin

- BRUISING; black eye. Swollen, purplish, pale, tender.
- Part FEELS COLD. Pains travel upward. Punctures.
- < HEAT, slight pressure, motion > COLD compresses.

LEDUM 38
Bruising

- Sharp WOUNDS: surgery, stabs, dental work. Falls.
- STITCHING, sore, tender. Neuralgia. Wounded pride.
- < Touch, motion, stretching, anger > Warmth, pressure.

STAPHYSAGRIA 53
Wounds

- Effects of head & brain injury: concussion, epilepsy, confusion, memory loss, irritability, depression, pain.
- Spine and low back injury. < REST > Motion, rubbing.

NAT SULPH 41
Head Injury

- EYE injury, splinters. Puncture wounds, falls, blows.
- Fever, pain, tenderness, inflammation after *surgery*.
- ANXIETY. SHOCK from injury, operation. Head injury.

ACONITUM 1
Eye - Surgery

- HEMORRHAGE. Wounds, cuts, bruises, nosebleed.
- Injury to VEINS, eye, ovaries. *Chronic effects of trauma.*
- Stops bleeding, removes pain, promotes healing.

HAMAMELIS
Wounds

- HEMORRHAGE from wounds or *internal injuries.*
- Bleeding from lungs, bladder, nose. B*right red blood.*
- Effects of falls, overexertion, after surgery, childbirth.

MILLEFOLIUM
Hemorrhage

5

SCAR TISSUE

THE SITUATION

We have an invisible framework that supports all of our tissues. Specialized cells called fibroblasts create elaborate webs of collagen fibers, which form an ultrafine network that sheaths and intertwines every fiber of our body, down to the cell itself. An extension of this connective tissue world, scar tissue occurs as a natural, essential part of ongoing repair. It adds structural strength to damaged areas of tissue, keeping the form and function of organs intact. Yet scar tissue can easily build up excessively, after a serious inflammation, or from subtle layering up of microscarring from ongoing trauma, repeated strain, and overuse.

More than 200 different homeopathic remedies act on scar tissue in various ways. Some prevent excess scar formation from occurring, ensuring the build-up of healthy connective tissue. Others can dissolve adhesions in or on various parts of the body. Others are for pain, infection, inflammation, or malignant processes that occur in areas of scar. Scar therapy has a longevity effect: elasticity is youth, while brittle connective tissue, wrinkling, and sagging flesh are aging. Most scar remedies also strengthen connective tissue, even helping in cases of cellulite.

Old-time naturopaths, acupuncturists, and other holistic practitioners have long known of the "toxic" effect of scars. Emotional memory resides *in the body*, directly in organs and tissues; Scars particularly retain negative biological and psychological experience. Aberrant information held within scars sends out neurological "static," which has far-reaching effects on other functions, tissues, and the mind itself,.and often need to be neutralized through techniques as diverse as Rolfing, laser acupuncture, Flower Essences, or homeopathy.

BODY LANGUAGE

• Scar tissue directly translates as fixation, rigidity, limitation, a part of oneself being frozen in a non-functional tissue matrix.

• Scars act as a badge of courage, honor, or "toughness," expressed by cosmetic adornment with scars (Aboriginal or African practices, or contemporary body piercing).

• Scar face = Deformity and wounding as a sign of strength, individuality.

• Scars signify being beaten up, damaged, wounded: scarred for life, scar on her soul. As the ultimate expression of form, we are defined by our scars and by how we respond to the challenge of our traumatic experiences.

• Scars can offer protection, a hiding place for walled-off toxic experience.

SCAR TISSUE

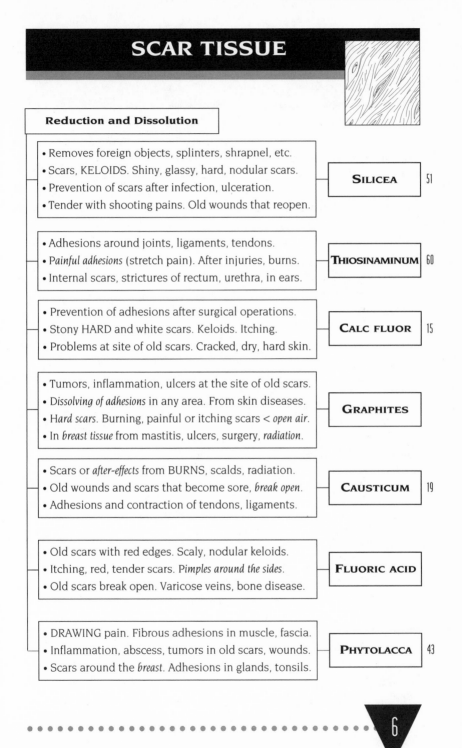

Reduction and Dissolution

- Removes foreign objects, splinters, shrapnel, etc.
- Scars, KELOIDS. Shiny, glassy, hard, nodular scars.
- Prevention of scars after infection, ulceration.
- Tender with shooting pains. Old wounds that reopen.

SILICEA 51

- Adhesions around joints, ligaments, tendons.
- *Painful adhesions* (stretch pain). After injuries, burns.
- Internal scars, strictures of rectum, urethra, in ears.

THIOSINAMINUM 60

- Prevention of adhesions after surgical operations.
- Stony HARD and white scars. Keloids. Itching.
- Problems at site of old scars. Cracked, dry, hard skin.

CALC FLUOR 15

- Tumors, inflammation, ulcers at the site of old scars.
- *Dissolving of adhesions* in any area. From skin diseases.
- *Hard scars.* Burning, painful or itching scars < *open air.*
- In *breast tissue* from mastitis, ulcers, surgery, *radiation.*

GRAPHITES

- Scars or *after-effects* from BURNS, scalds, radiation.
- Old wounds and scars that become sore, *break open.*
- Adhesions and contraction of tendons, ligaments.

CAUSTICUM 19

- Old scars with red edges. Scaly, nodular keloids.
- Itching, red, tender scars. *Pimples around the sides.*
- Old scars break open. Varicose veins, bone disease.

FLUORIC ACID

- DRAWING pain. Fibrous adhesions in muscle, fascia.
- Inflammation, abscess, tumors in old scars, wounds.
- Scars around the *breast.* Adhesions in glands, tonsils.

PHYTOLACCA 43

6

THE HUMAN SPINE

THE SITUATION

- The spine consists of four main curvatures: the neck, thorax, low back (lumbar), and the solid sacrum, with transition areas between the alternating curves, each with their own unique type and range of motion.
- The spine provides balance, support and mobility, and erect posture.
- The spine must be flexible, yet also maintain a stable center of gravity.
- The functional unit of the spine is the vertebrae, with its ligaments and joints, intervertebral discs, and the nerves that exit from the spine.
- Commonly, pain is produced when the small spinal joints are jammed and inflamed, caused by a combination of repeated stress, misuse, injury, poor or imbalanced posture, and chronic muscular tension.
- Damage to the disc can result in a bulge or rupture (they do not "slip"), which can compress the nerve, but nerve pain is often caused by tissue or joint inflammation and swelling, which impinges on the narrow space where the nerves conveying sensation and stimulating motion exit from the spine.
- Disc thinning occurs with age or injury; Combined with spinal arthritis (spondylosis) pain and nerve irritation commonly result.

SOLUTIONS

In the following pages, effective remedies for Cervical, Thoracic, and Lumbar conditions are outlined. Additional medicines are listed in the Therapeutic Guide, including those for spinal curvature and spinal injury. Also consider the remedies in the Arthritis Charts.

BODY LANGUAGE

- A striking difference between human beings and other creatures on this planet is our uniquely erect posture. The upright spine expresses our ability to span the realms from earth to heaven, our birthright as custodians of the planet, and our potential as conscious beings.
- Lack of spinal flexibility can express psychological rigidity, excess responsibility, or excess protectiveness, seen in tense, spastic spinal muscles.
- Slumping forward, towards the earth, expresses defeat, death. Arching backward opens one up, expressing hope, curiosity, the embracing of life.
- The body is symmetrical, with a central pole. The spine expresses balance between right and left, male and female, dark and light energies.
- The bony spine is the canal for the spinal cord, the sheath of nerves that conducts impulses to and from the brain to all organs and tissues, acting like a flexible steel cable housing the most delicate electrical wiring.

SPINAL AFFINITY

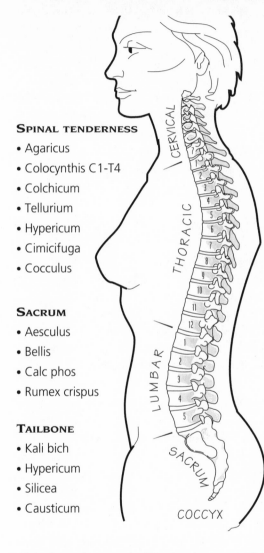

SPINAL TENDERNESS
- Agaricus
- Colocynthis C1-T4
- Colchicum
- Tellurium
- Hypericum
- Cimicifuga
- Cocculus

SACRUM
- Aesculus
- Bellis
- Calc phos
- Rumex crispus

TAILBONE
- Kali bich
- Hypericum
- Silicea
- Causticum

CERVICAL SPINE
- Gelsemium
- Lachnantes
- Calc phos
- Causticum
- Colocynthis

THORACIC SPINE
- Cimicifuga T1, T2
- Colocynthis T1-T4
- Tellurium T1-T5
- Ranunculus T3-T4
- Pulsatilla T5-T6
- Chelidonium T5-T7
- Agaricus T8-L2

LUMBAR SPINE
- Berberis L1-L3
- Bryonia L3-L4
- Pulsatilla L4
- Chelidonium L4-L5
- Nux vomica L5

This chart shows remedies that have an affinity to a specific area of the spine. The final choice of remedy is, of course, based on all symptoms and modalities. Consult the Condition Charts and Therapeutic Guide for additional information.

THE CERVICAL SPINE (NECK)

THE SITUATION

Neck pain is the second most common medical complaint, next to low back pain. The anatomy and movement of the neck are complex, providing a wide range of motion that allows great freedom to the sense organs of the head. Injury, poor posture, and chronic tension are the causes of most neck problems, though this area is also a common site for rheumatism, arthritis, and disc problems. Any of these conditions can cause nerve compression with pain radiating to the arms (*brachial neuralgia*), head, chest, or down the back. Pain between or beside the shoulder blades is often referred from the lower cervical spine. As we become overwhelmed with the sensory and emotional overload we experience day to day, stiffness and tension inexorably build up in the neck and shoulder area.

SOLUTIONS

- Structural alignment (spinal manipulation) of the neck has a well-known track record in rehabilitating acute and chronic neck problems.
- Homeopathy enhances this process, stimulating repair and healing.
- Many remedies deal with neck problems, ranging from inflammation, tension, and "stiff neck," to disc problems and nerve compression.
- In acute trauma, such as whiplash, the remedies in the Trauma Charts (especially Arnica and Rhus tox) are the first choice.
- The sixteen remedies in the following charts cover most other possibilities, and also help to change underlying patterns of muscle tension.

BODY LANGUAGE

- The first vertebra, the Atlas, holds up the globe of the head, allowing it free mobility to scan the environment, to hear, to see, and to experience. The neck is a mobile stalk with which we venture out into the world.
- The neck allows us to look up or down, expressing both hope or fear, confidence or despair. A stiff neck can express resistance to seeing.
- It is the conduit for all nourishment: food in the throat, air in the windpipe, and sensory experience and volition via the spinal cord.
- As the seat of the thyroid, the throat represents creativity and expression.
- The neck expresses grace, beauty, courage (head held high), nobility, pride.
- The neck is the bridge between head and heart, mind and hand.
- Many people "live in their head," cut off from the body at the neck.
- Constriction of the neck blocks our intake, our energy, our creativity. It is a two- way traffic jam, not letting experience in and / or expression out.
- We may be hung, decapitated, strangled, choked. Life is a "pain in the neck."

CERVICAL SPINE 1

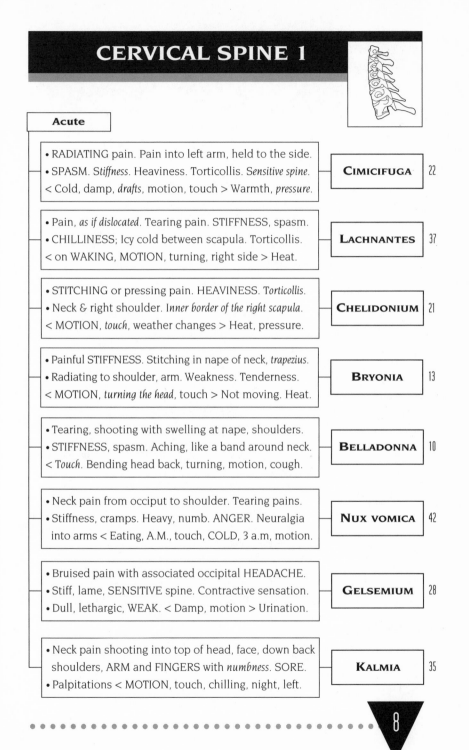

Acute

• RADIATING pain. Pain into left arm, held to the side. • SPASM. *Stiffness*. Heaviness. Torticollis. *Sensitive spine.* < Cold, damp, *drafts*, motion, touch > Warmth, *pressure.*	**CIMICIFUGA**	22
• Pain, *as if dislocated*. Tearing pain. STIFFNESS, spasm. • CHILLINESS; Icy cold between scapula. Torticollis. < on WAKING, MOTION, turning, right side > Heat.	**LACHNANTES**	37
• STITCHING or pressing pain. HEAVINESS. *Torticollis.* • Neck & right shoulder. *Inner border of the right scapula.* < MOTION, *touch*, weather changes > Heat, pressure.	**CHELIDONIUM**	21
• Painful STIFFNESS. Stitching in nape of neck, *trapezius.* • Radiating to shoulder, arm. Weakness. Tenderness. < MOTION, *turning the head*, touch > Not moving. Heat.	**BRYONIA**	13
• Tearing, shooting with swelling at nape, shoulders. • STIFFNESS, spasm. Aching, like a band around neck. < *Touch*. Bending head back, turning, motion, cough.	**BELLADONNA**	10
• Neck pain from occiput to shoulder. Tearing pains. • Stiffness, cramps. Heavy, numb. ANGER. Neuralgia into arms < Eating, A.M., touch, COLD, 3 a.m, motion.	**NUX VOMICA**	42
• Bruised pain with associated occipital HEADACHE. • Stiff, lame, SENSITIVE spine. Contractive sensation. • Dull, lethargic, WEAK. < Damp, motion > Urination.	**GELSEMIUM**	28
• Neck pain shooting into top of head, face, down back shoulders, ARM and FINGERS with *numbness*. SORE. • Palpitations < MOTION, touch, chilling, night, left.	**KALMIA**	35

8

CERVICAL SPINE 2

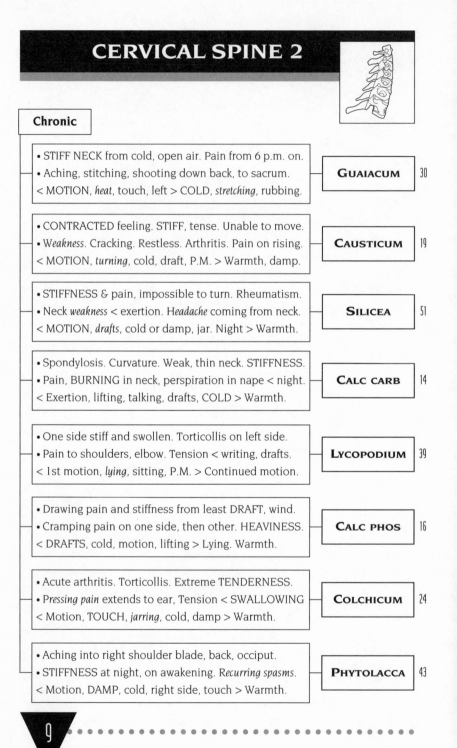

Chronic

• STIFF NECK from cold, open air. Pain from 6 p.m. on. • Aching, stitching, shooting down back, to sacrum. < MOTION, *heat*, touch, left > COLD, *stretching*, rubbing.	**GUAIACUM**	30
• CONTRACTED feeling. STIFF, tense. Unable to move. • *Weakness*. Cracking. Restless. Arthritis. Pain on rising. < MOTION, *turning*, cold, draft, P.M. > Warmth, damp.	**CAUSTICUM**	19
• STIFFNESS & pain, impossible to turn. Rheumatism. • Neck *weakness* < exertion. *Headache* coming from neck. < MOTION, *drafts*, cold or damp, jar. Night > Warmth.	**SILICEA**	51
• Spondylosis. Curvature. Weak, thin neck. STIFFNESS. • Pain, BURNING in neck, perspiration in nape < night. < Exertion, lifting, talking, drafts, COLD > Warmth.	**CALC CARB**	14
• One side stiff and swollen. Torticollis on left side. • Pain to shoulders, elbow. Tension < writing, drafts. < 1st motion, *lying*, sitting, P.M. > Continued motion.	**LYCOPODIUM**	39
• Drawing pain and stiffness from least DRAFT, wind. • Cramping pain on one side, then other. HEAVINESS. < DRAFTS, cold, motion, lifting > Lying. Warmth.	**CALC PHOS**	16
• Acute arthritis. Torticollis. Extreme TENDERNESS. • *Pressing pain* extends to ear, Tension < SWALLOWING < Motion, TOUCH, *jarring*, cold, damp > Warmth.	**COLCHICUM**	24
• Aching into right shoulder blade, back, occiput. • STIFFNESS at night, on awakening. *Recurring spasms*. < Motion, DAMP, cold, right side, touch > Warmth.	**PHYTOLACCA**	43

9

THE THORACIC SPINE

THE SITUATION

The twelve vertebrae of this area curve outward (kyphosis), placed strategically between the two inward curves of the neck and low back. Mechanically, the upper and lower ends of the thoracic spine are particularly subject to stress, as is the center of this convex curve. The thoracic spine is an intrinsic part of the rib "cage," aptly named as the housing for the lungs and heart, both as protection and as an auxiliary pump for breathing and voluntary inhalation and exhalation.

Muscle groups attach the shoulder blade to the vertebrae on one end and the arm on the other, making the thoracic spine an integral part of shoulder function. Thus, this part of the back receives stress from spinal posture and movement, rib and diaphragm motion, stress transmitted from the upper limbs and shoulders, and reflex neurological tension from the heart and lungs. Long periods working bent over and poor posture add to the insult. Besides pain syndromes, tension, and rib strains, the thoracic spine tends towards rigidity, with a loss of flexibility and the development of excess forward or sideways curves (scoliosis). Though a frequent site of muscular spasm and nagging pain, disc conditions rarely occur in this area. Pain produced in the rib / vertebra complex may radiate to the front of the body, at times mimicking heart or lung conditions. At the front the ribs are attached, via cartilage, to the breastbone, and these attachments are also subject to stiffness, soreness, or inflammation (costochondritis).

SOLUTIONS

Because of its transition location, many cervical spine remedies will help the upper thoracic spine, while lumbar spine remedies will be useful for the lower thoracic spine. Thoracic neuralgia, with pains radiating along the nerves to the chest, neck, or arms may require remedies found in the Sciatica Charts or in the appropriate section of the Therapeutic Guide.

BODY LANGUAGE

• The slumped posture of depression or the puffed-up chest of pride are due to changes in the thoracic spine, rather than other areas of the back.

• The thorax reflects changes in the heart more than any other musculoskeletal area: A poker-straight spine and tension may express mental rigidity, fear, resistance, or suspicion. An open heart is synonymous with relaxed musculature and a supple thoracic spine.

• Its anatomical and neurological relationship make the thorax subject to the physical and psychic stresses associated with the vulnerable breast area.

THORACIC SPINE

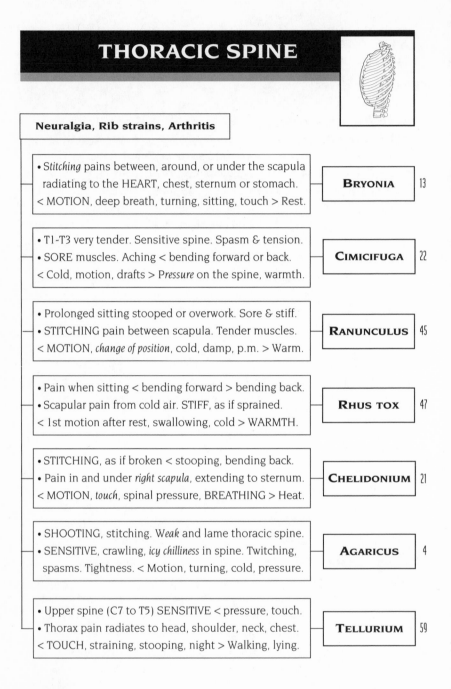

Neuralgia, Rib strains, Arthritis

- *Stitching* pains between, around, or under the scapula radiating to the HEART, chest, sternum or stomach. < MOTION, deep breath, turning, sitting, touch > Rest. — **BRYONIA** 13

- T1-T3 very tender. Sensitive spine. Spasm & tension.
- SORE muscles. Aching < bending forward or back. < Cold, motion, drafts > *Pressure* on the spine, warmth. — **CIMICIFUGA** 22

- Prolonged sitting stooped or overwork. Sore & stiff.
- STITCHING pain between scapula. Tender muscles. < MOTION, *change of position*, cold, damp, p.m. > Warm. — **RANUNCULUS** 45

- Pain when sitting < bending forward > bending back.
- Scapular pain from cold air. STIFF, as if sprained. < 1st motion after rest, swallowing, cold > WARMTH. — **RHUS TOX** 47

- STITCHING, as if broken < stooping, bending back.
- Pain in and under *right scapula*, extending to sternum. < MOTION, *touch*, spinal pressure, BREATHING > Heat. — **CHELIDONIUM** 21

- SHOOTING, stitching. *Weak* and lame thoracic spine.
- SENSITIVE, crawling, *icy chilliness* in spine. Twitching, spasms. Tightness. < Motion, turning, cold, pressure. — **AGARICUS** 4

- Upper spine (C7 to T5) SENSITIVE < pressure, touch.
- Thorax pain radiates to head, shoulder, neck, chest. < TOUCH, straining, stooping, night > Walking, lying. — **TELLURIUM** 59

LOW BACK PAIN

THE PROBLEM

Low back pain (LBP) is the most frequent disabling musculoskeletal condition. Eighty percent of people suffer from LBP in their life, resulting in 40 million days of lost work and a cost of $70 billion lost to the economy. Chronic poor posture is a major contributing factor. When the low back is held for prolonged periods in an arched-forward position (lordosis), great strain is put on the intervertebral discs, and the small joints of the spine are jammed together, causing inflammation (Facet Syndrome). Musculature tension, improper lifting, and poor nutritional status further weaken the tissues supporting the vertebrae. The lumbar spine is the primary area for gradual thinning and deterioration of the discs, or from an actual rupture or fragmentation of its outer fibers, resulting in extreme pain and possible nerve pressure. Spinal arthritis is common here with the formation of bony spurs or osteophytes. Additionally, trouble in major internal organs (the liver, uterus, kidney, etc.) have a reflex impact on the low back.

THE SOLUTION

- Homeopathy stimulates repair of tissue and promotes changes in the patterns of tension and stress. Improvement is accelerated by spinal manipulation, postural retraining, or the various types of bodywork or massage.
- There are many remedies for the lumbar spine, depending on the location, the acuteness or chronicity of the condition, and the exact symptoms and modalities experienced by the person.
- Fourteen common remedies for LBP are outlined in the following charts. In the case of injury, the remedies in the Trauma Charts are useful. For considerable pain in the legs, consult the Sciatica Charts. In more advanced cases of disc degeneration or arthrosis, consult the Arthritis Charts.

BODY LANGUAGE

- The low back is the *base* and root of our activity in the world. When we experience a loss of support or feel that challenges or responsibilities are too great, we simply "can't *stand* it." Rage, frustration, humiliation, or depression may be held in the low back, which is neurologically and psychologically associated with our "gut" feelings and deeper, suppressed instincts.
- The low back carries the most weight, and expresses the extent of the burden or load we bear, or if we feel overwhelmed and hopeless.
- The ability to adapt, withstand, or face up to stress or perceived onslaughts is expressed in the back; e.g. being spineless, having one's back against the wall, getting one's back up, oh my aching back!

LOW BACK 1

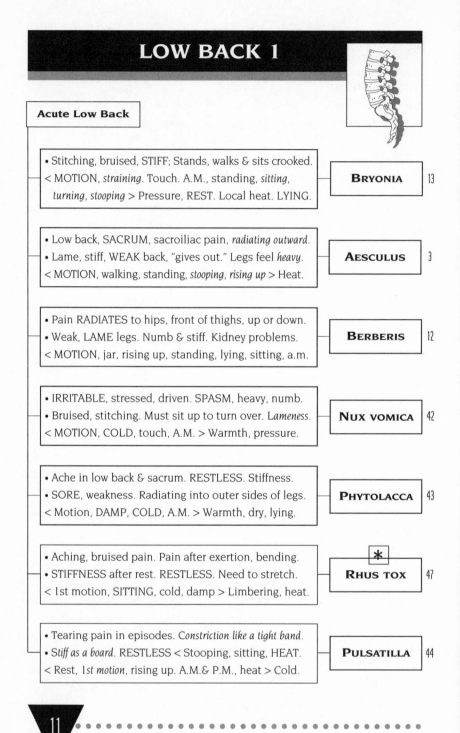

Acute Low Back

- Stitching, bruised, STIFF; Stands, walks & sits crooked.
- < MOTION, *straining*. Touch. A.M., standing, *sitting*, *turning, stooping* > Pressure, REST. Local heat. LYING.

BRYONIA   13

- Low back, SACRUM, sacroiliac pain, *radiating outward*.
- Lame, stiff, WEAK back, "gives out." Legs feel *heavy*.
- < MOTION, walking, standing, *stooping, rising up* > Heat.

AESCULUS   3

- Pain RADIATES to hips, front of thighs, up or down.
- Weak, LAME legs. Numb & stiff. Kidney problems.
- < MOTION, jar, rising up, standing, lying, sitting, a.m.

BERBERIS   12

- IRRITABLE, stressed, driven. SPASM, heavy, numb.
- Bruised, stitching. Must sit up to turn over. *Lameness*.
- < MOTION, COLD, touch, A.M. > Warmth, pressure.

NUX VOMICA   42

- Ache in low back & sacrum. RESTLESS. Stiffness.
- SORE, weakness. Radiating into outer sides of legs.
- < Motion, DAMP, COLD, A.M. > Warmth, dry, lying.

PHYTOLACCA   43

- Aching, bruised pain. Pain after exertion, bending.
- STIFFNESS after rest. RESTLESS. Need to stretch.
- < 1st motion, SITTING, cold, damp > Limbering, heat.

[*]
RHUS TOX   47

- Tearing pain in episodes. *Constriction like a tight band*.
- *Stiff as a board*. RESTLESS < Stooping, sitting, HEAT.
- < Rest, 1st motion, rising up. A.M.& P.M., heat > Cold.

PULSATILLA   44

11   •

LOW BACK 2

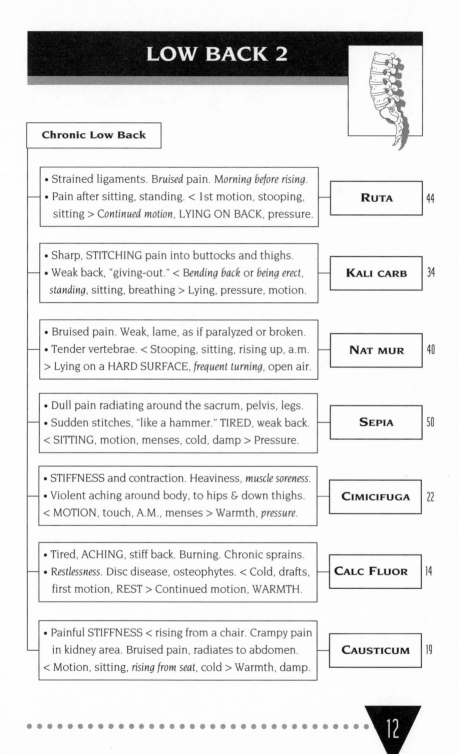

Chronic Low Back

- Strained ligaments. *Bruised* pain. *Morning before rising.*
- Pain after sitting, standing. < 1st motion, stooping, sitting > *Continued motion*, LYING ON BACK, pressure.

RUTA   44

- Sharp, STITCHING pain into buttocks and thighs.
- Weak back, "giving-out." < *Bending back* or *being erect, standing*, sitting, breathing > Lying, pressure, motion.

KALI CARB   34

- Bruised pain. Weak, lame, as if paralyzed or broken.
- Tender vertebrae. < Stooping, sitting, rising up, a.m. > Lying on a HARD SURFACE, *frequent turning*, open air.

NAT MUR   40

- Dull pain radiating around the sacrum, pelvis, legs.
- Sudden stitches, "like a hammer." TIRED, weak back. < SITTING, motion, menses, cold, damp > Pressure.

SEPIA   50

- STIFFNESS and contraction. Heaviness, *muscle soreness.*
- Violent aching around body, to hips & down thighs. < MOTION, touch, A.M., menses > Warmth, *pressure.*

CIMICIFUGA   22

- Tired, ACHING, stiff back. Burning. Chronic sprains.
- *Restlessness.* Disc disease, osteophytes. < Cold, drafts, first motion, REST > Continued motion, WARMTH.

CALC FLUOR   14

- Painful STIFFNESS < rising from a chair. Crampy pain in kidney area. Bruised pain, radiates to abdomen. < Motion, sitting, *rising from seat*, cold > Warmth, damp.

CAUSTICUM   19

12

SCIATICA (AND NEURALGIA)

THE SITUATION

The sciatic nerve is composed of branches from the lumbar and sacral spine, forming a thick bundle that provides nerve pathways to the entire leg, both for sensation and muscle function. Compression of this nerve can be caused by disc protrusion ("slipped disc"), or from arthritic spurs impinging on the nerve fibers. More common is simple compression of one or more nerve roots where they exit from the spine, caused by mis-alignments, joint inflammation, and swelling that narrows this small channel. The nerve itself and its fibrous linings can become inflamed, causing a true neuritis.

Depending on which vertebra is involved, pain will travel down specif-ic areas of the *back* of the leg, with possible spasm and weakness of the related muscles. Other abnormal sensations, like numbness, can occur. If nerve roots of the upper lumbar spine are affected, this causes similar types of symptoms in areas and muscles in the *front* of the leg. The treat-ment for this "lumbar neuralgia" is the same as that of sciatica.

With actual disc prolapse or herniation, with sudden onset from a minor movement, pain can be excruciating. Treatment consists of spinal manipulation or other bodywork, bed rest and / or traction, plus the ben-efits of homeopathy and nutritional supplements. Surgery is only indicat-ed if bladder or bowel function becomes disturbed, indicating spinal cord compression, or if chronic nerve pressure and persistent pain fail to be relieved by expert conservative care. This only happens in a small minori-ty of cases.

SOLUTIONS

Besides the remedies included here for nerve pain (neuralgia) and nerve inflammation (neuritis), all the remedies discussed in the three Low Back Charts may be applicable.

BODY LANGUAGE

- Sciatica is the proverbial "pain in the butt," involving a suppressed kick, a nagging underlying anger and frustration that is not being resolved, expressed, or acknowledged. "My leg is killing me" is a graphic expression of the projection of external stress onto a part of one's own body.
- Sciatica is not only painful, but prevents even the simplest act of locomo-tion, walking, sitting comfortably, or getting in and out of a car.
- It expresses an inability to go forward, a double-bind, feeling crippled.

SCIATICA 1

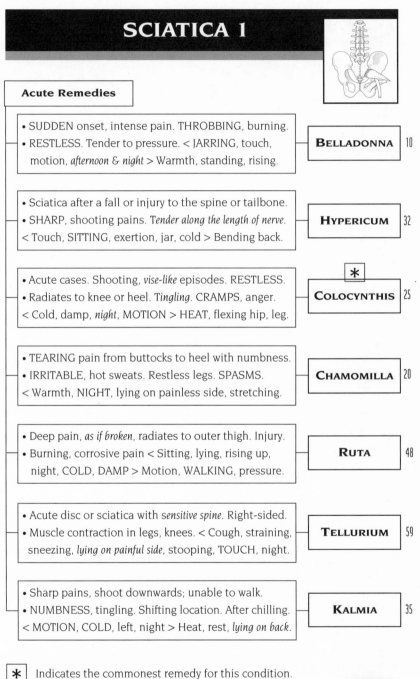

Acute Remedies

- SUDDEN onset, intense pain. THROBBING, burning.
- RESTLESS. Tender to pressure. < JARRING, touch, motion, *afternoon & night* > Warmth, standing, rising.

BELLADONNA 10

- Sciatica after a fall or injury to the spine or tailbone.
- SHARP, shooting pains. *Tender along the length of nerve.* < Touch, SITTING, exertion, jar, cold > Bending back.

HYPERICUM 32

- Acute cases. Shooting, *vise-like* episodes. RESTLESS.
- Radiates to knee or heel. *Tingling.* CRAMPS, anger. < Cold, damp, *night*, MOTION > HEAT, flexing hip, leg.

*

COLOCYNTHIS 25

- TEARING pain from buttocks to heel with numbness.
- IRRITABLE, hot sweats. Restless legs. SPASMS. < Warmth, NIGHT, lying on painless side, stretching.

CHAMOMILLA 20

- Deep pain, *as if broken*, radiates to outer thigh. Injury.
- Burning, corrosive pain < Sitting, lying, rising up, night, COLD, DAMP > Motion, WALKING, pressure.

RUTA 48

- Acute disc or sciatica with *sensitive spine*. Right-sided.
- Muscle contraction in legs, knees. < Cough, straining, sneezing, *lying on painful side*, stooping, TOUCH, night.

TELLURIUM 59

- Sharp pains, shoot downwards; unable to walk.
- NUMBNESS, tingling. Shifting location. After chilling. < MOTION, COLD, left, night > Heat, rest, *lying on back*.

KALMIA 35

| * | Indicates the commonest remedy for this condition.

13

SCIATICA 2

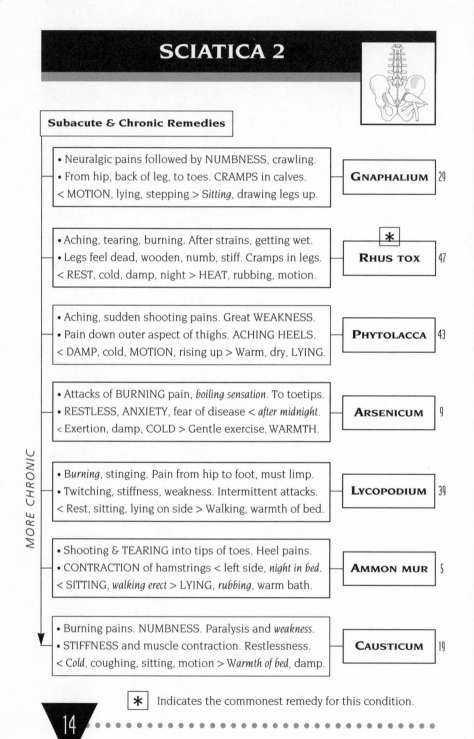

Subacute & Chronic Remedies

MORE CHRONIC

- Neuralgic pains followed by NUMBNESS, crawling.
- From hip, back of leg, to toes. CRAMPS in calves.
  < MOTION, lying, stepping > *Sitting*, drawing legs up.

GNAPHALIUM | 29

- Aching, tearing, burning. After strains, getting wet.
- Legs feel dead, wooden, numb, stiff. Cramps in legs.
  < REST, cold, damp, night > HEAT, rubbing, motion.

*
RHUS TOX | 47

- Aching, sudden shooting pains. Great WEAKNESS.
- Pain down outer aspect of thighs. ACHING HEELS.
  < DAMP, cold, MOTION, rising up > Warm, dry, LYING.

PHYTOLACCA | 43

- Attacks of BURNING pain, *boiling sensation*. To toetips.
- RESTLESS, ANXIETY, fear of disease < *after midnight*.
  < Exertion, damp, COLD > Gentle exercise, WARMTH.

ARSENICUM | 9

- *Burning*, stinging. Pain from hip to foot, must limp.
- Twitching, stiffness, weakness. Intermittent attacks.
  < Rest, sitting, lying on side > Walking, warmth of bed.

LYCOPODIUM | 39

- Shooting & TEARING into tips of toes. Heel pains.
- CONTRACTION of hamstrings < left side, *night in bed*.
  < SITTING, *walking erect* > LYING, *rubbing*, warm bath.

AMMON MUR | 5

- Burning pains. NUMBNESS. Paralysis and *weakness*.
- STIFFNESS and muscle contraction. Restlessness.
  < *Cold*, coughing, sitting, motion > *Warmth of bed*, damp.

CAUSTICUM | 19

---

* Indicates the commonest remedy for this condition.

14

THE EXTREMITIES

THE SITUATION

Like a five-pointed star, the limbs and head stretch out from our central trunk. The legs put us in touch with the earth, while the arms allow us to contact and change our world, to manipulate it for ill or good. In the center the head — and heart — decide what direction we take. The upper and lower limbs are built on the same template, with significant variation based on their very different needs. The upper limb is designed for flexibility, with a minimum of stability. The lower limbs maximize stability and forego flexibility. The ankle and wrist, the knee and elbow, the shoulder and hip are analogues of each other. Yet the shoulder is the loosest joint and the hip the most firmly attached.

Flexion is the process of bending a joint in, towards the body, while extension moves the joint outwards and away form the center. The upper and lower limbs are reverse images: The arms flex in, to the front of the body, and the legs flex in towards the back. We begin life in the fully flexed, fetal position. We assume this posture in sleep and again finally in death. This position represents maximum entropy, where everything is turned inward upon itself. All energy in internalized while all outward expression ceases. In extending our body, we literally reach for the stars, spread our wings, or move to the four corners of the globe. The hands can be the greatest source of creativity or instruments of destruction. The immense range of "flexibility" and mobility shown by the limbs is an appropriate mirror of the spectrum of human potential. Pain, limitation and disease in the limbs always has some connection to the meanings discussed above. The extremities and the voice are our prime channels for interacting with the world, both giving to it and receiving from it.

REMEDIES

Remedies have their own unique capacity to affect inflammation, swelling, stiffness, pain. Each has a unique set of symptoms and modalities which define their definitive character and their area of usefulness. Some remedies are known to affect the larger joints (shoulder, knee, ankle) or smaller joints (hands and feet, small joints of the spine), while others affect both. Specific remedies have a greater affinity for the upper limbs or the lower limbs. Other are relevant to problems that travel from joint to joint, either randomly or in a specific pattern (from above downwards, etc.).

THE SHOULDER

THE PROBLEM

The shoulder forms a very shallow joint, only held to the body by ligaments and the tendons of the powerful "rotator cuff" group of muscles. The shoulder sacrifices stability for flexibility (opposite of the hip, its analog in the lower limbs) to allow for free positioning of the hands, and to lift, pull, and push in powerful ways. The shoulder is the most easily dislocated joint and is readily sprained or pulled from either sudden stretching or with long-term overuse. Almost continually in use, the ligaments and capsule of the shoulder can be torn and weakened over time. Inflammation of the joint (synovitis), bursa, and tendon often coexist, creating a recurrent problem. Chronic tendonitis and bursitis may cause adhesions and calcium deposits in the area. A "frozen shoulder" results when scar tissue, caused by chronic inflammation, prevents mobility of the shoulder joint.

We are all familiar with the level of tension held in the shoulder muscles. An inward roll of the shoulder (rounded shoulders) increases the stress and tension in the area, compressing nerves and blood vessels.

THE SOLUTION

Many of the rheumatic remedies (Arthritis Charts) are useful here. Pain that begins in the neck and radiates into the shoulder or arm may need remedies from the Cervical Spine Chart. In acute bursitis or synovitis consider Belladonna, Bryonia, Apis, and Kalmia. In chronic states also think of Guaiacum, Calcarea, and Colchicum. Ferrum metallicum is a useful shoulder remedy, but has few indications other those in the chart opposite. For adhesions in the shoulder, try the remedies in the Scar Tissue Chart for several months before resorting to surgical procedures.

BODY LANGUAGE

• Shoulders droop with failure and depression, or expand and puff up with pride, and accomplishment: "A weight on the shoulders," "shouldering a burden," "a chip on his shoulder," "raise up your arms to heaven."
• "Broad shoulders" express strength, power, and prowess for both men and women (Ursula Andress). Shoulders are padded for this effect, including the use of epaulettes in the military of all nations.
• Shoulder problems can mean a sense of impotency, disempowerment, feeling beaten; unable to raise a hand to help oneself or pull oneself up.
• Shoulders may express a need to push things away, or to grasp what is desired. We shrug when we let go, give up, or don't know what to do.

SHOULDER-ARM

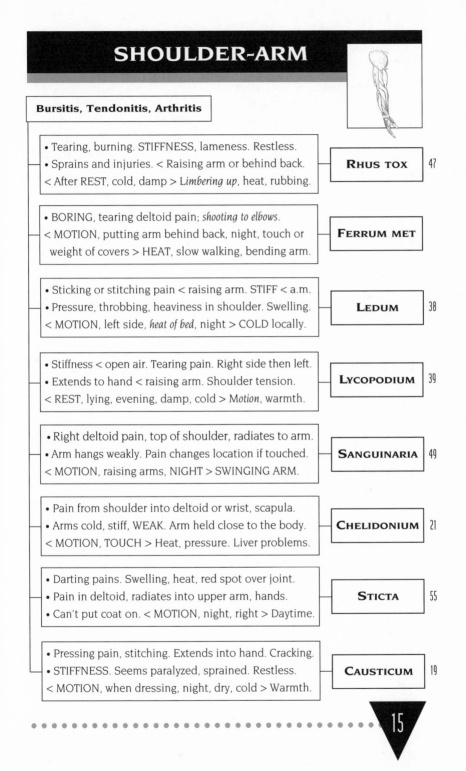

Bursitis, Tendonitis, Arthritis

- Tearing, burning. STIFFNESS, lameness. Restless.
- Sprains and injuries. < Raising arm or behind back.
< After REST, cold, damp > *Limbering up*, heat, rubbing.

RHUS TOX 47

- BORING, tearing deltoid pain; *shooting to elbows*.
< MOTION, putting arm behind back, night, touch or
  weight of covers > HEAT, slow walking, bending arm.

FERRUM MET

- Sticking or stitching pain < raising arm. STIFF < a.m.
- Pressure, throbbing, heaviness in shoulder. Swelling.
< MOTION, left side, *heat of bed*, night > COLD locally.

LEDUM 38

- Stiffness < open air. Tearing pain. Right side then left.
- Extends to hand < raising arm. Shoulder tension.
< REST, lying, evening, damp, cold > *Motion*, warmth.

LYCOPODIUM 39

- Right deltoid pain, top of shoulder, radiates to arm.
- Arm hangs weakly. Pain changes location if touched.
< MOTION, raising arms, NIGHT > SWINGING ARM.

SANGUINARIA 49

- Pain from shoulder into deltoid or wrist, scapula.
- Arms cold, stiff, WEAK. Arm held close to the body.
< MOTION, TOUCH > Heat, pressure. Liver problems.

CHELIDONIUM 21

- Darting pains. Swelling, heat, red spot over joint.
- Pain in deltoid, radiates into upper arm, hands.
- Can't put coat on. < MOTION, night, right > Daytime.

STICTA 55

- Pressing pain, stitching. Extends into hand. Cracking.
- STIFFNESS. Seems paralyzed, sprained. Restless.
< MOTION, when dressing, night, dry, cold > Warmth.

CAUSTICUM 19

15

THE WRIST

THE PROBLEM

Through its eight small carpal bones, articulating with the radius and ulna, the wrist is a network of interlacing ligaments and long tendons reaching down from the arm. It provides a flexible and adaptable platform for the subtle manipulations and fine movements of the hand. The wrist takes tremendous stress, particularly from holding the hands for long periods in a fixed position and from repetitive activities. Wrist sprains are common, and with almost constant use, the wrist is subject to osteoarthritis and is a favored site for rheumatoid arthritis. Thickening of the ligamentous bands can cause compression (carpal tunnel syndrome) with neuralgia, muscle weakness, and atrophy.

THE SOLUTION

Sprains of the wrist require Arnica or Bellis, usually followed by Rhus tox. For chronic effects of strains, Ruta and Calc carb are useful. Carpal tunnel syndrome: any remedy here or in the Therapeutic Guide. Ruta rapidly cures wrist ganglia (also Calc carb or fluor, Silica, Rhus). Ruta, Lycopodium, and Viola odorata are particularly suitable to the right wrist, while Guaiacum affects the left side more strongly. For weak wrists consider Ruta and others in the Therapeutic Guide. Because it is a favored site for rheumatoid arthritis and osteoarthritis, many remedies in the Arthritis Charts (particularly Arthritis Chart 4) may be beneficial for the wrist, as well as Silicea and Sulphur.

BODY LANGUAGE

- The wrist provides flexibility, adaptability, and freedom to be creative.
- Wrist problems indicate a loss of sense of control or creative ability.
- Criminals or captives are shackled, tied up, hand-cuffed at the wrist.
- Applying a "wrist lock" in Aikido or Judo incapacitates the opponent.
- Wrist problems are often a result of overstrain; many wrist remedies have symptoms of intense weariness and exhaustion, indicating that the person cannot "handle it" anymore.
- A "limp wrist" may express a lack of will or force. Energy flows freely through the straight wrist: in order to strike or point the wrist is straightened.
- In deformity or contracture of the wrist, the grotesque shape formed by the wrist is a striking image of contracted, suppressed life force.
- The wrist expresses grace, flow, relaxation. Rigid people always keep their wrists very stiff, not supple. We tighten the wrist in anger.
- Bracelets represent power, status (Rolex watch), attainment.

WRST

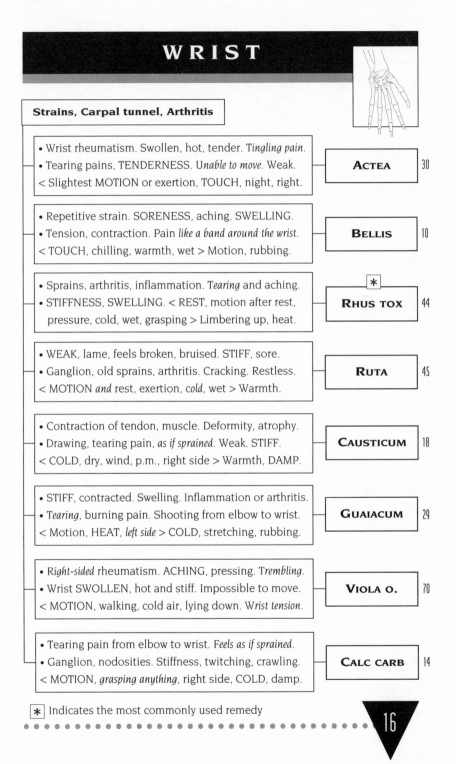

Strains, Carpal tunnel, Arthritis

- Wrist rheumatism. Swollen, hot, tender. *Tingling pain.*
- Tearing pains, TENDERNESS. *Unable to move.* Weak.
- < Slightest MOTION or exertion, TOUCH, night, right.

ACTEA 30

- Repetitive strain. SORENESS, aching. SWELLING.
- Tension, contraction. Pain *like a band around the wrist.*
- < TOUCH, chilling, warmth, wet > Motion, rubbing.

BELLIS 10

- Sprains, arthritis, inflammation. *Tearing* and aching.
- STIFFNESS, SWELLING. < REST, motion after rest, pressure, cold, wet, grasping > Limbering up, heat.

*

RHUS TOX 44

- WEAK, lame, feels broken, bruised. STIFF, sore.
- Ganglion, old sprains, arthritis. Cracking. Restless.
- < MOTION *and* rest, exertion, *cold*, wet > Warmth.

RUTA 45

- Contraction of tendon, muscle. Deformity, atrophy.
- Drawing, tearing pain, *as if sprained.* Weak. STIFF.
- < COLD, dry, wind, p.m., right side > Warmth, DAMP.

CAUSTICUM 18

- STIFF, contracted. Swelling. Inflammation or arthritis.
- *Tearing*, burning pain. Shooting from elbow to wrist.
- < Motion, HEAT, *left side* > COLD, stretching, rubbing.

GUAIACUM 29

- *Right-sided* rheumatism. ACHING, pressing. *Trembling.*
- Wrist SWOLLEN, hot and stiff. Impossible to move.
- < MOTION, walking, cold air, lying down. W*rist tension.*

VIOLA O. 70

- Tearing pain from elbow to wrist. *Feels as if sprained.*
- Ganglion, nodosities. Stiffness, twitching, crawling.
- < MOTION, *grasping anything*, right side, COLD, damp.

CALC CARB 14

* Indicates the most commonly used remedy

16

THE HIP JOINT

THE PROBLEM

Designed for weight-bearing, the hip joint is an intrinsic part of walking, and stands up well to the stress put upon it. A true ball and socket, straddled by strong ligamentous bands, the hip is the most tightly fitting joint of the body, moved by the powerful muscles of the buttock and thigh. The analog of the shoulder in the upper limb, the hip joint has sacrificed relative mobility for stability. It flexes, extends, rotates, and draws in or out. Yet, unlike the shoulder, any movement of the hip affects the whole limb.

Pain in the hip can be due to muscle tension, inflamed ligaments, or inflammation of the joint lining itself. "Hip" pain is often actually referred from problems in the low back or sciatic nerve. Osteoarthritis is the most common and serious cause of hip pain, with no true inflammation, but a gradual deterioration of the cartilage. Typically, pain begins on standing or sitting (weight-bearing), and progresses to pain on motion (walking), to finally, pain even when at rest. Hip pain will often be felt in the side of the thigh, or may radiate into the buttocks, thighs, or down the side of the leg.

SOLUTIONS

Since injury is a major cause for development of hip arthrosis, trauma remedies are important for complete healing and prevention of damage. Colocynthis, the main remedy for acute sciatica, is also necessary in many acute hip problems. Along with the medicines indicated here, those in the Arthritis Charts may be called for. The Therapeutic Guide lists other homeopathics for hip arthritis and arthrosis, including Bryonia, Sepia, Calc carb, or Phosphorus.

BODY LANGUAGE

• The grace and timing of the remarkable human feat of upright walking is largely due to the rhythmic action of the hip and sacroiliac joints, in balancing the forces of gravity and muscular action.

• The pelvic girdle is directly associated with the womb, sexuality, fertility, and creative forces. It is the transfer point between earthly energies and upper, solar, emotional forces. It expresses their balance.

• Just in front of the sacrum lies the body's center of gravity for weight-bearing and the pelvic chakra or "hara." In Eastern traditions this is considered the center of physical prowess and of the life force itself.

• Weight around the hips is like a protective barrier or padding.

• Hip lameness expresses a loss of grace, prowess, sexuality or sensuality, the ability to stand up for oneself, or to contain a creative center.

HIP JOINT

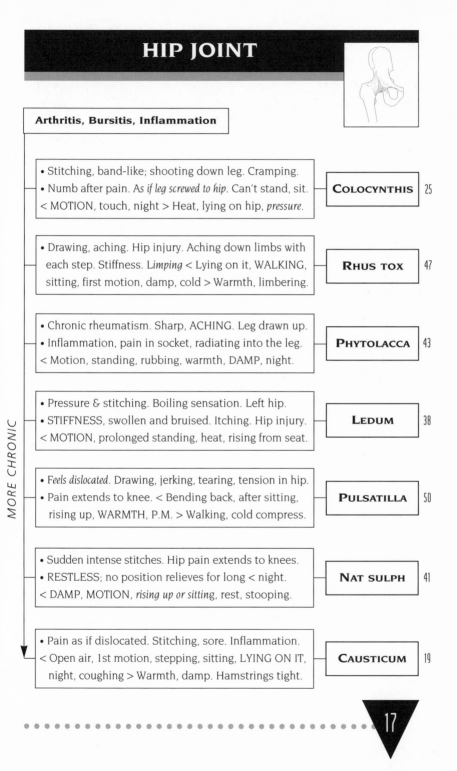

Arthritis, Bursitis, Inflammation

- Stitching, band-like; shooting down leg. Cramping.
- Numb after pain. *As if leg screwed to hip.* Can't stand, sit.
< MOTION, touch, night > Heat, lying on hip, *pressure.*

COLOCYNTHIS | 25

- Drawing, aching. Hip injury. Aching down limbs with each step. Stiffness. *Limping* < Lying on it, WALKING, sitting, first motion, damp, cold > Warmth, limbering.

RHUS TOX | 47

- Chronic rheumatism. Sharp, ACHING. Leg drawn up.
- Inflammation, pain in socket, radiating into the leg.
< Motion, standing, rubbing, warmth, DAMP, night.

PHYTOLACCA | 43

- Pressure & stitching. Boiling sensation. Left hip.
- STIFFNESS, swollen and bruised. Itching. Hip injury.
< MOTION, prolonged standing, heat, rising from seat.

LEDUM | 38

- *Feels dislocated.* Drawing, jerking, tearing, tension in hip.
- Pain extends to knee. < Bending back, after sitting, rising up, WARMTH, P.M. > Walking, cold compress.

PULSATILLA | 50

- Sudden intense stitches. Hip pain extends to knees.
- RESTLESS; no position relieves for long < night.
< DAMP, MOTION, *rising up or sitting*, rest, stooping.

NAT SULPH | 41

- Pain as if dislocated. Stitching, sore. Inflammation.
< Open air, 1st motion, stepping, sitting, LYING ON IT, night, coughing > Warmth, damp. Hamstrings tight.

CAUSTICUM | 19

MORE CHRONIC

17

KNEE CONDITIONS

THE PROBLEM

With its shallow joint surface, moon-shaped cartilages (menisci), ligaments on each side, and internal ligaments (cruciates), the knee is highly susceptible to twisting injuries, sprains, and strains. It is also famous for being slow to heal and recovering poorly. It is subject to inflammatory joint disease, including synovitis, bursitis, and rheumatoid arthritis. Other conditions can affect the kneecap (chondromalacia) and the tendon attachments (osteochondrosis). Repeated wear and strain tend the knee towards osteoarthritis later on. Symptoms include swelling, popping, grinding, giving way, locking, instability, loss of motion, and muscle wasting.

SOLUTIONS

Though we are taught that cartilage can never regenerate and only scars after injury, clinical experience and recent research show otherwise. Nutritional and homeopathic therapy can promote tissue healing and reverse serious joint changes, helping the body to regenerate cartilage.

Acute Care

• Acute remedies for the knee reduce inflammation, swelling, and pain, accelerating the healing of injured joint structures. Remedies in the Trauma Chart should be used, with Arnica as the first remedy for injury, often followed by Rhus tox.

• Apis is remarkable for swelling of the knee (bursitis, etc.).

Chronic Care

• For arthritis of the knee, consult the Arthritis Charts that follow.

• An effective regimen for many stubborn knee problems is the following: Ruta 6c morning and night, with the tissue salts, Calc fluor 6x, Silicea 6x, and Calc phos 6x, taken together, three times daily (apart from the Ruta). After one month, the Ruta can be increased to the 12c strength, twice daily. Later, Ruta 30c or 30x can be used once daily.

BODY LANGUAGE

• The knee expresses the ability to stand upright, to assert one's independence, strength, and power, or to lose all this and more.

• The knee moves in only one plane — back and forth: it is a polarity of yes or no, either independence or submission (voluntary or forced).

• "On bended knees," "brought to his knees," "crawling on hands and knees." "You must crawl before you can walk."

• On our knees we pledge loyalty, we pray, are knighted, are enslaved.

KNEE

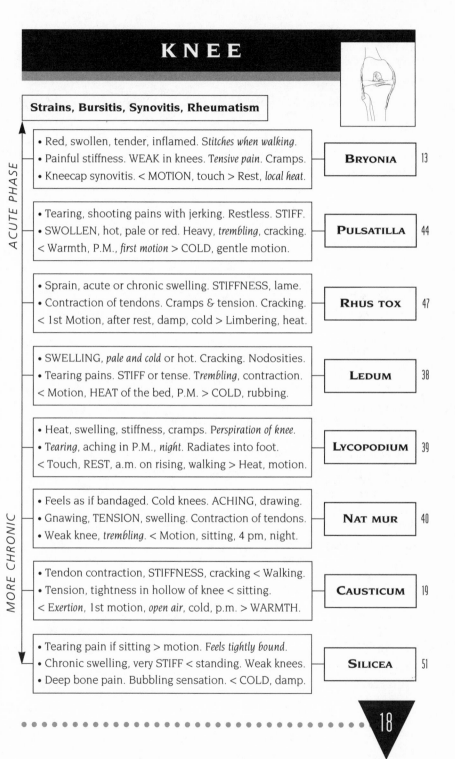

Strains, Bursitis, Synovitis, Rheumatism

ACUTE PHASE

- Red, swollen, tender, inflamed. *Stitches when walking.*
- Painful stiffness. WEAK in knees. *Tensive pain.* Cramps.
- Kneecap synovitis. < MOTION, touch > Rest, *local heat.*

BRYONIA 13

- Tearing, shooting pains with jerking. Restless. STIFF.
- SWOLLEN, hot, pale or red. Heavy, *trembling*, cracking.
- < Warmth, P.M., *first motion* > COLD, gentle motion.

PULSATILLA 44

- Sprain, acute or chronic swelling. STIFFNESS, lame.
- Contraction of tendons. Cramps & tension. Cracking.
- < 1st Motion, after rest, damp, cold > Limbering, heat.

RHUS TOX 47

- SWELLING, *pale and cold* or hot. Cracking. Nodosities.
- Tearing pains. STIFF or tense. *Trembling*, contraction.
- < Motion, HEAT of the bed, P.M. > COLD, rubbing.

LEDUM 38

- Heat, swelling, stiffness, cramps. *Perspiration of knee.*
- *Tearing*, aching in P.M., *night.* Radiates into foot.
- < Touch, REST, a.m. on rising, walking > Heat, motion.

LYCOPODIUM 39

MORE CHRONIC

- Feels as if bandaged. Cold knees. ACHING, drawing.
- Gnawing, TENSION, swelling. Contraction of tendons.
- Weak knee, *trembling.* < Motion, sitting, 4 pm, night.

NAT MUR 40

- Tendon contraction, STIFFNESS, cracking < Walking.
- Tension, tightness in hollow of knee < sitting.
- < *Exertion*, 1st motion, *open air*, cold, p.m. > WARMTH.

CAUSTICUM 19

- Tearing pain if sitting > motion. *Feels tightly bound.*
- Chronic swelling, very STIFF < standing. Weak knees.
- Deep bone pain. Bubbling sensation. < COLD, damp.

SILICEA 51

ANKLE CONDITIONS

THE PROBLEM

The 26 bones of the foot are designed to bear the weight of the body and transport it over all types of terrain. The tibia and fibula of the leg sit firmly on the talus bone of the foot, supported strongly by multiple bands of ligaments on each side. Designed mainly as a pivot mechanism for backward and forward movement, the ankle complex also allows the foot to turn inward or outward. It is easily injured by turning or twisting in a lateral direction, such that ankle spain the most common orthopedic condition. Recurrent sprains of varying severity result in tearing, overstretching, and weakening of the ankle ligaments, making the joint less stable. The joint is then prone to adhesions and arthritic changes. Anatomically, foot problems such as loss of the arch (pronation or "flat feet") naturally affect the ankle, pushing it off its stable base. Muscles, ligaments, and tendon are common sources of leg and ankle pain and dysfunction, including muscle pulls or "shin splints."

SOLUTIONS

- Muscle strains or ankle injury should be dealt with by remedies in the Trauma Charts, particularly Arnica and Rhus tox, followed by Ledum. Fractures or pulled tendons may require Ruta and Symphytum.
- Weak ankles can be strengthened by Calc carb, Calc phos, Calc fluor, Silicea, Ruta, etc. For arthritic changes, check the Arthritis Charts.
- Achilles tendonitis will generally respond to Cimicifuga or Strontium carb. Ruta is always useful if the tendon is injured or torn.
- For shin splints, Bellis is particularly effective, along with Bryonia, Rhus tox, and Ruta, depending on the specific symptom picture.
- Additional remedies are suggested in the Therapeutic Guide.

BODY LANGUAGE

- This simple joint, when sprained, has us incapacitated or "hobbled." The entire mobility of the body and ability to function is lost.
- Ankles have been considered an object of beauty: graceful, sexy, a place for anklets and jewelry. Flashing or showing of an ankle is seductive.
- Ankle problems can relate to an inability to go forward or carry on, feeling crippled, impeded. We are bound, shackled, put in irons, put in chains. A crutch is needed to just limp along.
- A suppressed desire to kick can result in a stiff, swollen and painful ankle, holding in the anger that could not be expressed.

ANKLE

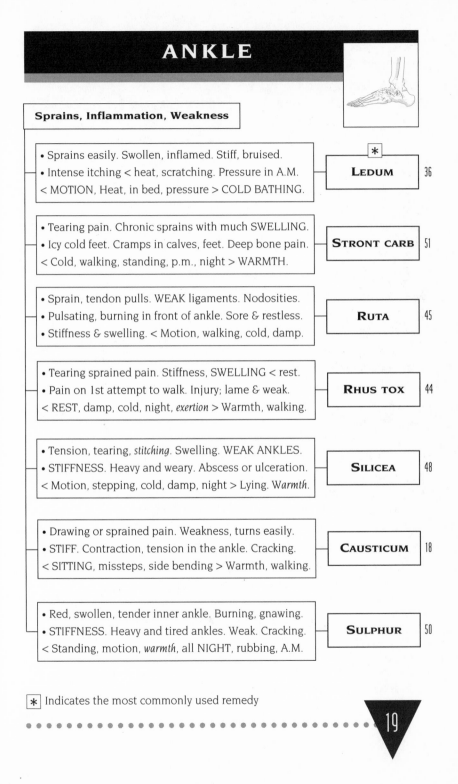

Sprains, Inflammation, Weakness

- Sprains easily. Swollen, inflamed. Stiff, bruised.
- Intense itching < heat, scratching. Pressure in A.M.
< MOTION, Heat, in bed, pressure > COLD BATHING.

[*] LEDUM 36

- Tearing pain. Chronic sprains with much SWELLING.
- Icy cold feet. Cramps in calves, feet. Deep bone pain.
< Cold, walking, standing, p.m., night > WARMTH.

STRONT CARB 51

- Sprain, tendon pulls. WEAK ligaments. Nodosities.
- Pulsating, burning in front of ankle. Sore & restless.
- Stiffness & swelling. < Motion, walking, cold, damp.

RUTA 45

- Tearing sprained pain. Stiffness, SWELLING < rest.
- Pain on 1st attempt to walk. Injury; lame & weak.
< REST, damp, cold, night, *exertion* > Warmth, walking.

RHUS TOX 44

- Tension, tearing, *stitching*. Swelling. WEAK ANKLES.
- STIFFNESS. Heavy and weary. Abscess or ulceration.
< Motion, stepping, cold, damp, night > Lying. *Warmth*.

SILICEA 48

- Drawing or sprained pain. Weakness, turns easily.
- STIFF. Contraction, tension in the ankle. Cracking.
< SITTING, missteps, side bending > Warmth, walking.

CAUSTICUM 18

- Red, swollen, tender inner ankle. Burning, gnawing.
- STIFFNESS. Heavy and tired ankles. Weak. Cracking.
< Standing, motion, *warmth*, all NIGHT, rubbing, A.M.

SULPHUR 50

[*] Indicates the most commonly used remedy

ARTHRITIS

THE PROBLEM

Arthritis is the number one chronic illness in America, affecting over 40 million people, including 285,000 children. One in seven individuals (15% of the population) have arthritis, two-thirds of these being women. For three million people arthritis severely limits everyday activity. Holistic medicine recognizes a multiplicity of causes for arthritis including diet, nutritional deficiencies, environmental toxins, a weakened immune system, joint stress, liver or intestinal toxicity (dysbiosis), and constitutional predispositions (*miasms*). Rheumatoid arthritis is an autoimmune condition with intense inflammation of the joints and progressive destruction of cartilage, tendons, and soft tissue. It accounts for 3% of all cases of arthritis. Osteoarthritis is a gradual erosion and deterioration of the joint cartilage. It occurs to a degree in all people with aging, but strongly affects over 16 million Americans, creating bone spurs and painful, stiff joints.

SOLUTIONS

A combination of natural therapies offers significant benefit for sufferers of arthritis, without the weakening effects of symptomatic drugs. Prognosis is based on the unique mix of variables that make up each case of arthritis. Remedies are prescribed for the symptoms which express this uniqueness.

Acute care

Acute remedies reduce inflammation, swelling and pain, sparing fragile connective tissue, nerves and blood vessels from further damage

Chronic care

Homeopathic medicines may halt further progression of arthritic disease. Further, deep-acting remedies are capable of altering existing pathology, returning elasticity, flexibility, and function to contracted tissue. *Constitutional remedies* improve overall immune, hepatic, and metabolic health.

BODY LANGUAGE

• The crippling nature of arthritis is graphic and striking.
• In the later stage of arthritis there is an inward contraction of the flexor tendons, pulling the person into a huddled, curled-up fetal position.
• The inward contraction of arthritis expresses severe repression, unresolved feeling, and suppression of the entire emotional life.
• The unresolved feelings can include internalized rage, terror, or grief.
• Touch, pressure, or the least contact with the joint (with the world) means pain. All movement — meaning all active living — is too painful.

ARTHRITIS 1

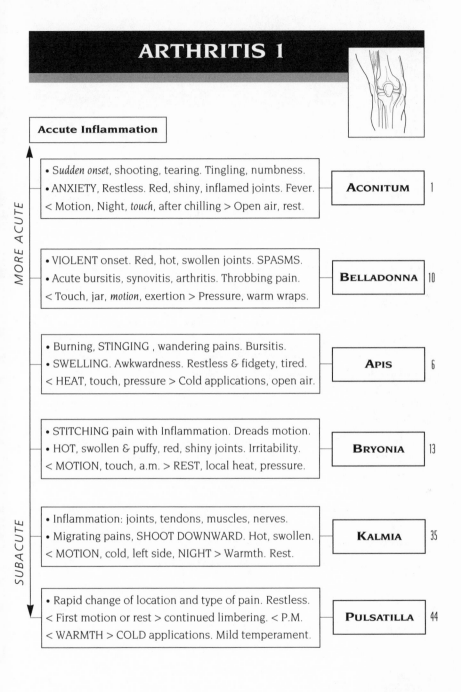

Accute Inflammation

MORE ACUTE

• *Sudden onset*, shooting, tearing. Tingling, numbness.
• ANXIETY, Restless. Red, shiny, inflamed joints. Fever.
< Motion, Night, *touch*, after chilling > Open air, rest.

ACONITUM   1

• VIOLENT onset. Red, hot, swollen joints. SPASMS.
• Acute bursitis, synovitis, arthritis. Throbbing pain.
< Touch, jar, *motion*, exertion > Pressure, warm wraps.

BELLADONNA   10

• Burning, STINGING , wandering pains. Bursitis.
• SWELLING. Awkwardness. Restless & fidgety, tired.
< HEAT, touch, pressure > Cold applications, open air.

APIS   6

• STITCHING pain with Inflammation. Dreads motion.
• HOT, swollen & puffy, red, shiny joints. Irritability.
< MOTION, touch, a.m. > REST, local heat, pressure.

BRYONIA   13

SUBACUTE

• Inflammation: joints, tendons, muscles, nerves.
• Migrating pains, SHOOT DOWNWARD. Hot, swollen.
< MOTION, cold, left side, NIGHT > Warmth. Rest.

KALMIA   35

• Rapid change of location and type of pain. Restless.
< First motion or rest > continued limbering. < P.M.
< WARMTH > COLD applications. Mild temperament.

PULSATILLA   44

20

ARTHRITIS 2

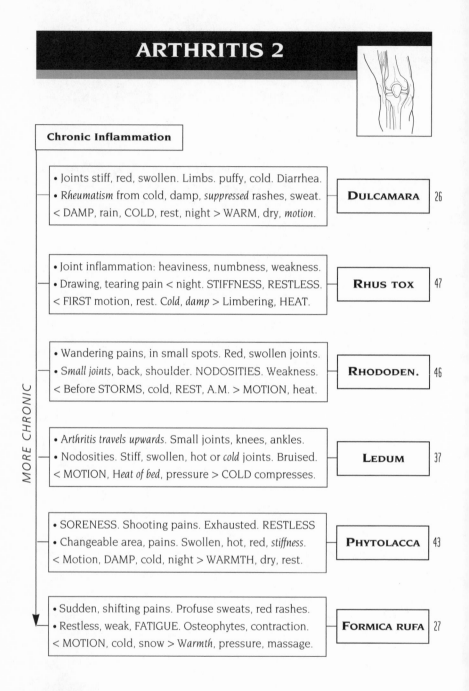

Chronic Inflammation

MORE CHRONIC

- Joints stiff, red, swollen. Limbs. puffy, cold. Diarrhea.
- *Rheumatism* from cold, damp, *suppressed* rashes, sweat.
< DAMP, rain, COLD, rest, night > WARM, dry, *motion*.

DULCAMARA | 26

- Joint inflammation: heaviness, numbness, weakness.
- Drawing, tearing pain < night. STIFFNESS, RESTLESS.
< FIRST motion, rest. *Cold, damp* > Limbering, HEAT.

RHUS TOX | 47

- Wandering pains, in small spots. Red, swollen joints.
- *Small joints*, back, shoulder. NODOSITIES. Weakness.
< Before STORMS, cold, REST, A.M. > MOTION, heat.

RHODODEN. | 46

- *Arthritis travels upwards.* Small joints, knees, ankles.
- Nodosities. Stiff, swollen, hot or *cold* joints. Bruised.
< MOTION, *Heat of bed*, pressure > COLD compresses.

LEDUM | 37

- SORENESS. Shooting pains. Exhausted. RESTLESS
- Changeable area, pains. Swollen, hot, red, *stiffness*.
< Motion, DAMP, cold, night > WARMTH, dry, rest.

PHYTOLACCA | 43

- Sudden, shifting pains. Profuse sweats, red rashes.
- Restless, weak, FATIGUE. Osteophytes, contraction.
< MOTION, cold, snow > *Warmth*, pressure, massage.

FORMICA RUFA | 27

21

INFLAMMATORY PHASE

The diagram below shows the spectrum of the common remedies used in the acute phase of joint inflammation, including synovitis and arthritis. The order is not to be considered rigid, but suggests the degree of chronicity or increasing depth and duration of symptoms.

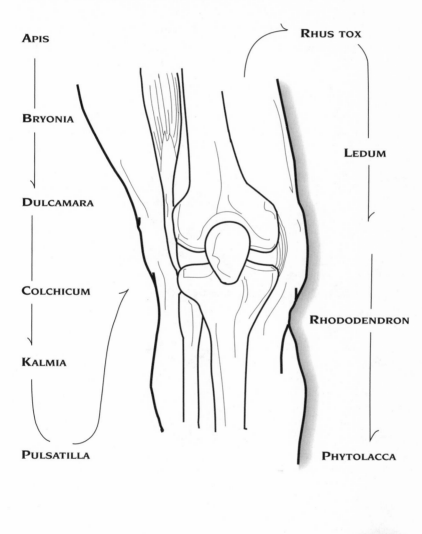

APIS

RHUS TOX

BRYONIA

LEDUM

DULCAMARA

COLCHICUM

RHODODENDRON

KALMIA

PULSATILLA

PHYTOLACCA

ARTHRITIS 3

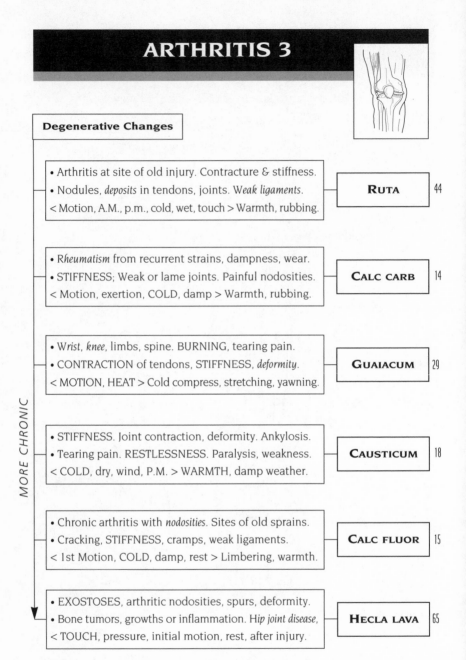

Degenerative Changes

- Arthritis at site of old injury. Contracture & stiffness.
- Nodules, *deposits* in tendons, joints. *Weak ligaments.*
< Motion, A.M., p.m., cold, wet, touch > Warmth, rubbing.

RUTA   44

- *Rheumatism* from recurrent strains, dampness, wear.
- STIFFNESS; Weak or lame joints. Painful nodosities.
< Motion, exertion, COLD, damp > Warmth, rubbing.

CALC CARB   14

- W*rist, knee,* limbs, spine. BURNING, tearing pain.
- CONTRACTION of tendons, STIFFNESS, *deformity.*
< MOTION, HEAT > Cold compress, stretching, yawning.

GUAIACUM   29

- STIFFNESS. Joint contraction, deformity. Ankylosis.
- Tearing pain. RESTLESSNESS. Paralysis, weakness.
< COLD, dry, wind, P.M. > WARMTH, damp weather.

CAUSTICUM   18

- Chronic arthritis with *nodosities.* Sites of old sprains.
- Cracking, STIFFNESS, cramps, weak ligaments.
< 1st Motion, COLD, damp, rest > Limbering, warmth.

CALC FLUOR   15

- EXOSTOSES, arthritic nodosities, spurs, deformity.
- Bone tumors, growths or inflammation. *Hip joint disease,*
< TOUCH, pressure, initial motion, rest, after injury.

HECLA LAVA   65

MORE CHRONIC

23

DEGENERATIVE PHASE

The remedies shown below are the core homeopathic medicines in degenerative joint conditions. Those on the left are involved with chronic inflammatory and sclerotic reactions. Those on the right represent deeper destruction or atrophy of soft tissue and bone, where active inflammation is no longer occurring to any degree.

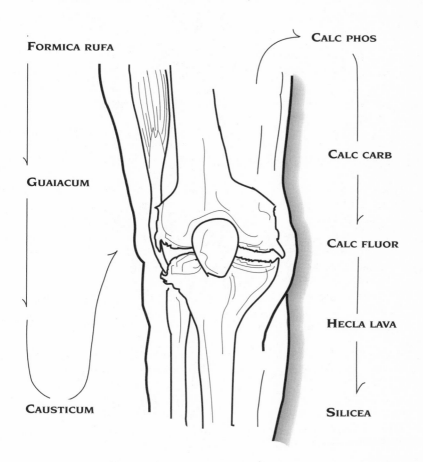

FORMICA RUFA

GUAIACUM

CAUSTICUM

CALC PHOS

CALC CARB

CALC FLUOR

HECLA LAVA

SILICEA

ARTHRITIS 4

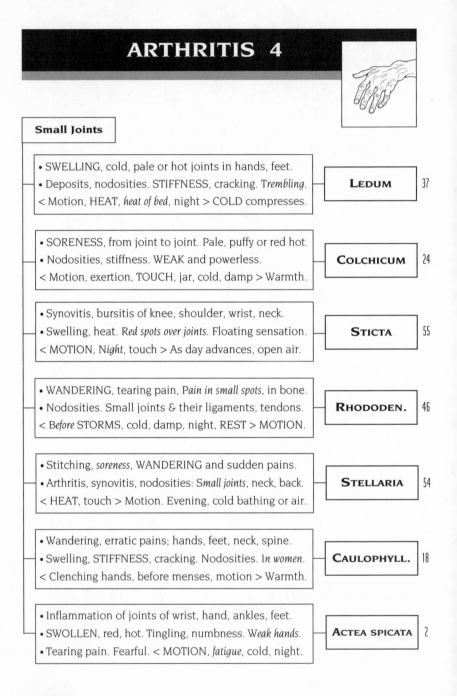

Small Joints

• SWELLING, cold, pale or hot joints in hands, feet. • Deposits, nodosities. STIFFNESS, cracking. *Trembling.* < Motion, HEAT, *heat of bed*, night > COLD compresses.	**LEDUM**	37
• SORENESS, from joint to joint. Pale, puffy or red hot. • Nodosities, stiffness. WEAK and powerless. < Motion, exertion, TOUCH, jar, cold, damp > Warmth.	**COLCHICUM**	24
• Synovitis, bursitis of knee, shoulder, wrist, neck. • Swelling, heat. *Red spots over joints.* Floating sensation. < MOTION, N*ight*, touch > As day advances, open air.	**STICTA**	55
• WANDERING, tearing pain, *Pain in small spots*, in bone. • Nodosities. Small joints & their ligaments, tendons. < *Before* STORMS, cold, damp, night, REST > MOTION.	**RHODODEN.**	46
• Stitching, *soreness*, WANDERING and sudden pains. • Arthritis, synovitis, nodosities: *Small joints*, neck, back. < HEAT, touch > Motion. Evening, cold bathing or air.	**STELLARIA**	54
• Wandering, erratic pains; hands, feet, neck, spine. • Swelling, STIFFNESS, cracking. Nodosities. *In women.* < Clenching hands, before menses, motion > Warmth.	**CAULOPHYLL.**	18
• Inflammation of joints of wrist, hand, ankles, feet. • SWOLLEN, red, hot. Tingling, numbness. *Weak hands.* • Tearing pain. Fearful. < MOTION, *fatigue*, cold, night.	**ACTEA SPICATA**	2

ARTHRITIS • SMALL JOINTS

HAND

Actea spicata
Calc carb
Causticum
Colchicum
Guaiacum
Kalmia
Ledum
Lycopodium
Rhus tox
Ruta

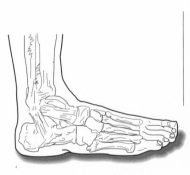

WRIST

Actea spicata
Calc carb
Caulophyllum
Guaiacum
Lachesis
Pulsatilla
Rhus tox
Ruta
Viola

FINGERS

Actea spicata • Calc carb • Calc fluor • Caulophyllum • Colchicum • Hecla
• Ledum • Phytolacca • Rhododendron • Rhus tox • Silicea.

ANKLE

Actea spicata
Caulophyllum
Guaiacum
Kalmia
Ledum
Lycopodium
Rhododendron
Ruta

FOOT

Causticum
Ledum
Guaiacum
Phytolacca
Rhododendron
Ruta

TOES

Actea spicata • Caulophyllum • Chelidonium • Guaiacum • Kalmia
• Ledum • Lycopodium • Pulsatilla • Rhododendron • Ruta

See the Therapeutic Guide for additional remedy choices.

26

FIBROMYALGIA (FMS)

THE PROBLEM

First described in 1843 as a type of rheumatism, "fibrositis" has only recently been recognized as a systemic disorder with far-reaching effects. An estimated 5% of people suffer from fibromyalgia, but the number is probably much greater since diagnosis is often difficult. There are no definitive laboratory tests, and symptoms are diverse and sometimes vague. Individuals may have been on a long, frustrating search for answers and relief. Fibromyalgia symptoms are centered around generalized fatigue and aching, and most sufferers experience panful, tender nodules in many of the 18 key areas that define this syndrome. These include shoulders, buttocks, occiput, upper chest, knees, and elbows. Other prominent symptoms include, insomnia, headache, cramps, irritable bowel syndrome, food allergies, weight gain, unusual sensations (paresthesias), low thyroid, depression, anxiety, irritability, and poor concentration. FMS may be linked to chronic fatigue syndrome, as there is a clear immunological dysfunction present. Other causes include sleep disorders, phosphorus deposits in the tissue, chemical or environmental sensitivities, and chronic viral, bacterial or parasitic infections.

SOLUTIONS

Because fibromyalgia is a broad metabolic or systemic disorder, in-depth cure requires constitutional prescribing by a homeopathic practitioner. A 1989 study published in the British Medical Journal verified the effectiveness of Rhus tox, showing favorable results and improvement of symptoms. The remedies suggested here are powerful aids in reducing connective tissue and muscle inflammation and associated pain and disability.

BODY LANGUAGE

• The pain experienced by people with fibromyalgia is widespread, changeable and debilitating, and in many cases is a precursor to osteoarthritis.

• This syndrome often expresses a life situation that is intolerable, painful, or unbearable. There is restriction on all sides with no escape.

• The effective remedies, like Cimicifuga, Rhus tox, and Causticum, all have symptoms of being too tight, constricted, trapped, and despairing.

• The fatigue and aching in key areas is crippling. Fibromyalgia patients may show a strong sense of being downtrodden or victimized; there may, be a history of strong emotional, verbal, or physical abuse.

• Other remedies related to prolonged emotional stress should be considered, including Nat mur, Lachesis, Ignatia, Arsenicum, and Staphysagria.

FIBROMYALGIA

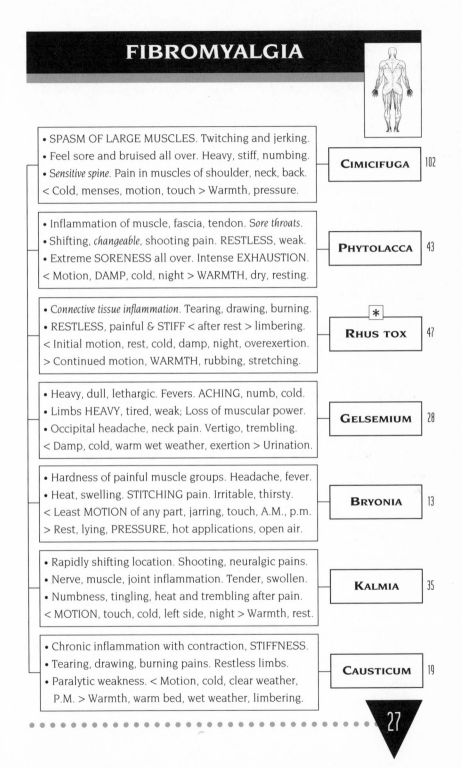

- SPASM OF LARGE MUSCLES. Twitching and jerking.
- Feel sore and bruised all over. Heavy, stiff, numbing.
- *Sensitive spine.* Pain in muscles of shoulder, neck, back.
< Cold, menses, motion, touch > Warmth, pressure.

CIMICIFUGA 102

- Inflammation of muscle, fascia, tendon. *Sore throats.*
- Shifting, *changeable*, shooting pain. RESTLESS, weak.
- Extreme SORENESS all over. Intense EXHAUSTION.
< Motion, DAMP, cold, night > WARMTH, dry, resting.

PHYTOLACCA 43

- *Connective tissue inflammation.* Tearing, drawing, burning.
- RESTLESS, painful & STIFF < after rest > limbering.
< Initial motion, rest, cold, damp, night, overexertion.
> Continued motion, WARMTH, rubbing, stretching.

*

RHUS TOX 47

- Heavy, dull, lethargic. Fevers. ACHING, numb, cold.
- Limbs HEAVY, tired, weak; Loss of muscular power.
- Occipital headache, neck pain. Vertigo, trembling.
< Damp, cold, warm wet weather, exertion > Urination.

GELSEMIUM 28

- Hardness of painful muscle groups. Headache, fever.
- Heat, swelling. STITCHING pain. Irritable, thirsty.
< Least MOTION of any part, jarring, touch, A.M., p.m.
> Rest, lying, PRESSURE, hot applications, open air.

BRYONIA 13

- Rapidly shifting location. Shooting, neuralgic pains.
- Nerve, muscle, joint inflammation. Tender, swollen.
- Numbness, tingling, heat and trembling after pain.
< MOTION, touch, cold, left side, night > Warmth, rest.

KALMIA 35

- Chronic inflammation with contraction, STIFFNESS.
- Tearing, drawing, burning pains. Restless limbs.
- Paralytic weakness. < Motion, cold, clear weather,
  P.M. > Warmth, warm bed, wet weather, limbering.

CAUSTICUM 19

27

HEADACHE

THE PROBLEM

Seventy per cent of the people get headaches, with 50 million visiting doctors annually! Today headaches are generally classified as *tension type* or *migraine type*, though current research indicates they may be different degrees of the same condition. This makes sense, since many of the effective homeopathic headache remedies can be used for either type. *The symptoms are the key.* Tension headaches account for 90% of headaches, with typical constrictive sensations, soreness, or painful knots in tense neck and scalp muscles. Migraine occurs in about 23 million Americans or about 9% of the population and affect women three times more than men. There may be an aura of visual lights, blurred vision, or tingling in *classic migraine*, or this may be absent (*common migraine*). Cluster headaches occur in intense episodes. There is a great deal of variety in headache symptoms, including severity, frequency, duration, location, and associated symptoms such as nausea and vomiting. Causes of headache include eyestrain, food allergies, hormonal imbalance, nutritional deficiencies, toxicity, digestive or intestinal disturbances, emotional stress, and altered serotonin levels.

SOLUTIONS

Conventional therapy merely consists of pain killers and palliative (symptomatic) treatment. Homeopathy is effective for acute headaches, and more importantly, has an excellent record in the affecting permanent cures. Different remedies are used for acute care, as opposed to long-term cure, the main point being the exact correspondence of the remedy picture with both the headache and the make-up of the individual.

BODY LANGUAGE

- The connotations of "head" as the seat of authority and power are obvious, yet in many cultures, the "mind" is considered to be the heart. Headache may thus indicate a preoccupation with our "head brain" and the neglect of our "feeling-intuitive" brains, or a conflict between the two.
- The "contents" of our head might be unbearable, due to guilt, shame, and self-hate. Migraine sufferers may not be living their true, heartfelt life.
- The tremendous internal pressures and conflicts that many people carry can be (temporarily) released through the "steam valve" of headaches.
- Many of our important headache remedies have strong components of suppressed or unexpressed emotions (grief, anger, fear, etc.).
- Sensory overload or sensitivity to what we see and hear can be a literal headache. Many head pains are descriptive of contraction, bursting, etc.

HEADACHE 1

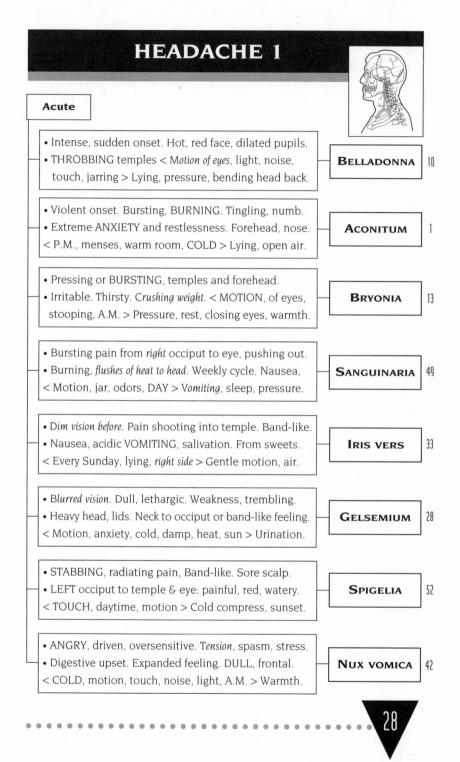

Acute

- Intense, sudden onset. Hot, red face, dilated pupils.
- THROBBING temples < *Motion of eyes*, light, noise, touch, jarring > Lying, pressure, bending head back.

BELLADONNA 10

- Violent onset. Bursting, BURNING. Tingling, numb.
- Extreme ANXIETY and restlessness. Forehead, nose. < P.M., menses, warm room, COLD > Lying, open air.

ACONITUM 1

- Pressing or BURSTING, temples and forehead.
- Irritable. Thirsty. *Crushing weight.* < MOTION, of eyes, stooping, A.M. > Pressure, rest, closing eyes, warmth.

BRYONIA 13

- Bursting pain from *right* occiput to eye, pushing out.
- Burning, *flushes of heat to head.* Weekly cycle. Nausea, < Motion, jar, odors, DAY > *Vomiting*, sleep, pressure.

SANGUINARIA 49

- *Dim vision before.* Pain shooting into temple. Band-like.
- Nausea, acidic VOMITING, salivation. From sweets. < Every Sunday, lying, *right side* > Gentle motion, air.

IRIS VERS 33

- *Blurred vision.* Dull, lethargic. Weakness, trembling.
- Heavy head, lids. Neck to occiput or band-like feeling. < Motion, anxiety, cold, damp, heat, sun > Urination.

GELSEMIUM 28

- STABBING, radiating pain, Band-like. Sore scalp.
- LEFT occiput to temple & eye: painful, red, watery. < TOUCH, daytime, motion > Cold compress, sunset.

SPIGELIA 52

- ANGRY, driven, oversensitive. *Tension*, spasm, stress.
- Digestive upset. Expanded feeling. DULL, frontal. < COLD, motion, touch, noise, light, A.M. > Warmth.

NUX VOMICA 42

28

HEADACHE 2

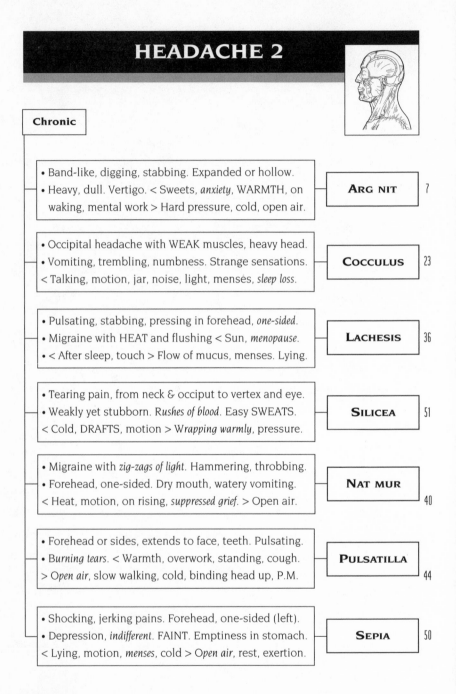

Chronic

- Band-like, digging, stabbing. Expanded or hollow.
- Heavy, dull. Vertigo. < Sweets, *anxiety*, WARMTH, on waking, mental work > Hard pressure, cold, open air.

ARG NIT   7

- Occipital headache with WEAK muscles, heavy head.
- Vomiting, trembling, numbness. Strange sensations. < Talking, motion, jar, noise, light, menses, *sleep loss*.

COCCULUS   23

- Pulsating, stabbing, pressing in forehead, *one-sided*.
- Migraine with HEAT and flushing < Sun, *menopause*.
- < After sleep, touch > Flow of mucus, menses. Lying.

LACHESIS   36

- Tearing pain, from neck & occiput to vertex and eye.
- Weakly yet stubborn. *Rushes of blood.* Easy SWEATS. < Cold, DRAFTS, motion > *Wrapping warmly*, pressure.

SILICEA   51

- Migraine with *zig-zags of light*. Hammering, throbbing.
- Forehead, one-sided. Dry mouth, watery vomiting. < Heat, motion, on rising, *suppressed grief.* > Open air.

NAT MUR   40

- Forehead or sides, extends to face, teeth. Pulsating.
- *Burning tears.* < Warmth, overwork, standing, cough. > *Open air*, slow walking, cold, binding head up, P.M.

PULSATILLA   44

- Shocking, jerking pains. Forehead, one-sided (left).
- Depression, *indifferent*. FAINT. Emptiness in stomach. < Lying, motion, *menses*, cold > Open air, rest, exertion.

SEPIA   50

29

HEADACHE LOCATIONS 1

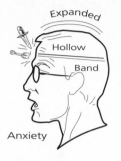

Expanded
Hollow
Band
Anxiety

ARGENTUM NIT

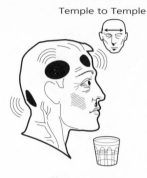

Temple to Temple

BELLADONNA

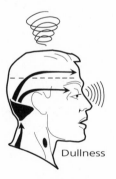

Bursting
Dry

BRYONIA

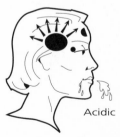

Weak   Heavy
Trembling

COCCULUS

Dullness

GELSEMIUM

Acidic

IRIS VERSICOLOR

30

HEADACHE LOCATIONS 2

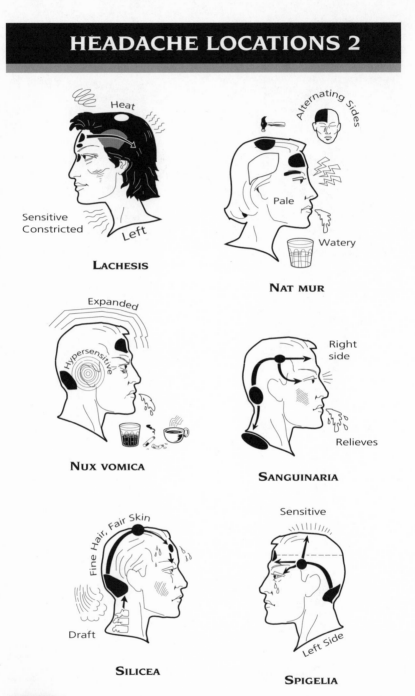

Heat

Sensitive
Constricted

Left

LACHESIS

Alternating Sides

Pale

Watery

NAT MUR

Expanded

Hypersensitive

NUX VOMICA

Right
side

Relieves

SANGUINARIA

Fine Hair, Fair Skin

Draft

SILICEA

Sensitive

Left Side

SPIGELIA

31

Materia Medica

MATERIA MEDICA INDEX

Usual name	Latin name	English name
1. Aconitum	*Aconitum napellus*	Monkshood
2 Actea	*Actea spicata*	Baneberry
3. Aesculus	*Aesculus hippocastanum*	Horse Chestnut
4. Agaricus	*Agaricus muscarius*	Fly Agaric
5. Ammonium mur	*Ammonium muriaticum*	Ammonium Chloride
6. Apis	*Apis mellifica*	Honeybee
7. Argentum nit	*Argentum nitricum*	Silver Nitrate
8. Arnica	*Arnica montana*	Leopard's Bane
9. Arsenicum	*Arsenicum album*	Oxide of Arsenic
10. Belladonna	*Atropa belladonna*	Deadly Nightshade
11. Bellis	*Bellis perennis*	Common Daisy
12. Berberis	*Berberis vulgaris*	Barberry
13. Bryonia	*Bryonia alba*	White Bryony
14. Calc carb	*Calcarea carbonica*	Calcium Carbonate
15. Calc fluor	*Calcarea fluorica*	Calcium Fluoride
16. Calc phos	*Calcarea phosphorica*	Calcium Phosphate
17. Calendula	*Calendula officinalis*	Marigold
18. Caulophyllum	*Caulophyllum thalictroides*	Blue Cohosh
19. Causticum	*Causticum Hahnemanni*	Potassium Hydrate
20. Chamomilla	*Matricaria chamomilla*	German Chamomile
21. Chelidonium	*Chelidonium majus*	Greater Celandine
22. Cimicifuga	*Cimicifuga racemosa*	Black Cohosh
23. Cocculus	*Cocculus indicus*	Indian Cockle
24. Colchicum	*Colchicum autumnale*	Meadow Saffron
25. Colocynthis	*Citrullus colocynthis*	Bitter Cucumber
26. Dulcamara	*Solanum dulcamara*	Bittersweet
27. Formica rufa	*Formica rufa*	Red Ants
28. Gelsemium	*Gelsemium sempervirens*	Yellow Jasmine
29. Gnaphalium	*Gnaphalium polycephalum*	Sweet Everlasting
30. Guaiacum	*Guaiacum officinale*	Lignum Vitae
31. Hecla lava	*Hecla lava*	Lava of Mt. Hecla
32. Hypericum	*Hypericum perforatum*	St. John's Wort
33. Iris	*Iris versicolor*	Blue Flag
34. Kali carb	*Kali carbonicum*	Potassium Carbonate
35. Kalmia	*Kalmia latifolia*	Mountain Laurel
36. Lachesis	*Lachesis muta*	Bushmaster Snake

Usual name	Latin name	English name
37. Lachnantes	*Lachnantes tinctoria*	Red Root
38. Ledum	*Ledum palustre*	Labrador Tea
39. Lycopodium	*Lycopodium clavatum*	Club Moss
40. Nat mur	*Natrum muriaticum*	Common Salt
41. Nat sulph	*Natrum sulphuricum*	Sodium Sulphate
42. Nux vomica	*Strychnos nux vomica*	Poison Nut
43. Phytolacca	*Phytolacca decandra*	Poke Root
44. Pulsatilla	*Pulsatilla nigricans*	Wind Flower
45. Ranunculus	*Ranunculus bulbosus*	Bulbous Buttercup
46. Rhododendron	*Rhododendron chrysanthum*	Yellow Snow Rose
47. Rhus tox	*Rhus toxicodendron*	Poison Ivy
48. Ruta	*Ruta graveolens*	Garden Rue
49. Sanguinaria	*Sanguinaria canadensis*	Blood Root
50. Sepia	*Sepia officinalis*	Ink of the Cuttlefish
51. Silicea	*Silicic acid*	Quartz Crystal
52. Spigelia	*Spigelia anthelmia*	Pinkroot
53. Staphysagria	*Delphinium Staphysagria*	Larkspur
54. Stellaria	*Stellaria media*	Chickweed
55. Sticta	*Sticta pulmonaria*	Lungwort
56. Strontium carb	*Strontium carbonicum*	Strontium Carbonate
57. Sulphur	*Sulphur sublimatum*	Sulphur (Brimstone)
58. Symphytum	*Symphytum officinalis*	Comfrey
59. Tellurium	*Tellurium*	Tellurium
60. Thiosinaminum	*Allyl sulphocarbamide*	Oil of Mustard Seed
61. Viola	*Viola odorata*	Sweet Violet

ACONITUM

Monkshood

▼ KEYNOTES

➤ Sudden intense pains with burning, tingling, numbness.
➤ Inflammation: Acute arthritis. Acute neuralgia. Acute headache.
➤ ANXIETY, restlessness. < Motion, night, touch, COLD.

▼ MUSCULOSKELETAL SYMPTOMS

Pain
- SUDDEN, violent, acute onset. Shooting pains.
- Intense, unbearable pain. TEARING, cutting or bruised.
- *Burning* pain. Bursting, pulsating. Like boiling water.
- TINGLING and *numbness*, especially in the extremities. Heaviness.

Causes
- COLD. *Chilling.* Cold *drafts* or *winds.* Injuries or surgery. Heat. Sun.
- Frights, shock (ailment dates back to a terrifying experience).
- Suppression of nasal discharge or *suppressed perspiration.*

Locations
- JOINTS: Inflamed; Bright red, shiny, *swollen*, sensitive to touch with fevers, warm sweats which relieve symptoms. Cracking of joints. Weak ligaments.
- Arthritis of large joints: shoulders, ankles, elbow, knee, wrist.
- *Headache*: Forehead, root of nose to vertex, above eye. *Facial neuralgia.*
- *Back*: Numb, STIFF, BRUISED feeling. Tearing pains in neck, low back or between scapulae. Formication up and down the back.
- *Extremities*: Neuralgia. Limbs feel lame, bruised.
  Tearing pains < motion, touch.

Associated
- Trembling, twitching, NUMBNESS, TINGLING.
- RESTLESSNESS, tossing about, which gives no relief.
- DRY, HOT skin. Intense thirst for cold water.
- HOT HANDS, COLD FEET.
- Face red, hot, swollen, *flushed, but pales on rising.* Nosebleed.
- HEAVINESS. Swollen feelings. Weary and exhausted.
- ANXIETY; worry, anguish. *Fear of imminent death.*

ACONITUM NAPELLUS

Modalities

< NIGHT, evening. TOUCH. N*oise, music, light.*
< Getting CHILLED. Warm room. Heat of the sun. Before menses.
< Motion, lying on the affected side, rising up, *right side.* Mental work.
> Open air, *sitting still,* sweating. Lying with the head high.

▼ SYMPTOM PROFILE

Psychological

• Extreme anxiety, *fear of death,* of the future, of *crowds,* dark, suffocation. Claustrophobia. Agoraphobia. Anxiety about one's health.
• Illness originating in a frightening experience or trauma.
• FEAR AFTER ACCIDENTS, *earthquakes.* Nightmares. E*asily startled.*
• Hyperventilation. Confused and disoriented with headaches.

Metabolic

• Acute onset conditions: People requiring Aconitum generally have a strong constitution, vitality, or reactive ability.
• Inflammation or first stage of acute upper respiratory conditions (flu, colds, bronchitis, etc.) with heat and dryness of eyes, skin, throat, nose, mouth and intense thirst. Acute hypertension.
• FAINTNESS: from pain, fear, hysteria.
• Antidoted by wines, coffee, lemonade, acid fruit.

▼ DOSAGE

Potency

• 6th to 10M.
• Some feel that the 6th is best for headache, 12th and higher for accidents. Higher potencies for neuralgias or emotional states.

Repetition

• Repeat frequently (hourly) in acute conditions.
• Generally used as an acute, short-acting remedy, though Vithoulkas and others now suggest it is a deep-acting constitutional remedy.

▼ CLINICAL CONDITIONS

• Anxiety or fear after trauma • Arthritis (acute stages)
• Facial Neuralgia • Headache • Neuralgic pain • Rheumatic fever
• Rheumatoid arthritis • SHOCK • Trauma.

ACTEA

Baneberry

▼ KEYNOTES

➤ Arthritis of the small joints; wrists, fingers, ankles, feet.
➤ Tearing pain. SWELLING, tingling. WEAK, lame joints, limbs.
➤ < SLIGHT EXERTION, MOTION, fatigue, cold, touch, night.

▼ MUSCULOSKELETAL SYMPTOMS

Pain

• Tearing and tingling pains. Subacute or chronic conditions.

Location

• Small joints in general: of the hand, *fingers*. Distal phalanges.
• WRIST, ankles and feet. Also knee and sacrum.

Associated

• SWELLING < after exertion. Motion becomes impossible.
• WEAKNESS of hand, arm or other affected parts.
• TINGLING sensations. *Numbness* of hands, feet, etc.
• Rheumatism from suppressed foot sweat.
• Deformity; enlargement and stiffness of joints (chronic cases).

Modalities

< MOTION. After walking. *Touch*. Pressure.
< SLIGHT FATIGUE or EXERTION causes swelling, weakness, pain.
< COLD. Change of weather. Open air (weakness, pain).
< Night. *Right side*. After a fright. In men (more than women).
> Morning.

Specific Joints

• *Wrist*: SWOLLEN, red, hot, intense pain. Weak. Unable to move it.
• *Hands*: Weak, as if paralyzed. Arms feel lame. Intense pain in palm
  on pressure. Fingers cold, numb, discolored.
• *Knee*: Pain, weariness. Trembling of thighs when lifting them. Weak-
  ness of legs < change of temperature.
• *Foot joints*: Swollen after walking.
• *Sacrum*: Bruised, sore pain < lying on the side.
• *Low back* pain, like a hot iron.

ACTEA SPICATA

▼ **SYMPTOM PROFILE**

Psychological

- FEAR OF DEATH, at night in bed, when alone. Fear of and sense of failure. Fear of insanity. Anxiety < lying or at rest > motion.
- Desires company < when alone.
- Depressed, gloomy, hopeless with weeping.
- Confusion, absent-minded, delirium. Indecision. Unable to do any mental work, though he desires to. Alcoholism.

Metabolic

- WEAKNESS. Lassitude after *talking*, eating, *walking in the open air*.
- Actea spicata more common for men; Caulophyllum for women.
- CHILLY. Often useful in older people.
- *Shortness of breath* < in the fresh air.

Digestive System

- Loss of appetite. Effects of taking spoiled food, bad fruit.
- Cramps, stomach pain with sour vomiting. Liver congestion.

Head

- Throbbing headache on the *vertex* of the head, radiating to area *between the eyes* < night, walking > open air. Vertigo with headache.
- Crushing pain in left frontal area.
- Goose bumps on the head. Itching scalp alternating with heat.
- Warm sweat on the head. Pimples on the scalp.
- Headaches caused by coffee (but coffee may also relieve).
- Pain in upper jaw, cheekbone, radiating to the temples.

▼ **DOSAGE**

Potency

- Mainly the 3x and 3c have been used, but 6, 12, or 30 are effective.

Repetition

- May be repeated daily for several weeks in lower potencies.

▼ **CLINICAL CONDITIONS**

- Arthritis • Dental neuralgia • Facial neuralgia • Gout • Headache
- Rheumatism • Wrist conditions (carpal tunnel syndrome, etc.).

AESCULUS

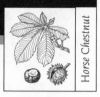

Horse Chestnut

▼ KEYNOTES

➤ Dull ache in the sacrum, sacroiliac, low back. Radiating pains.
➤ WEAKNESS, stiffness, heaviness. Hemorrhoids / varicose veins.
➤ < WALKING, motion, STOOPING, rising up, morning > Heat.

▼ LOW BACK SYMPTOMS

Pain

• Dull, ACHING, CONSTANT back pain. Tearing pain on walking.
• RADIATING, flying, shooting along nerves.
• *Changeable*, wandering pains.

Location

• Sacroiliac, SACRUM, hip, lumbosacral joints, pubic symphysis.
• Starts in back or sacrum and radiates to hips, etc.

Associated

• WEAKNESS of back: "Gives out." Paralytic feeling.
• LAMENESS, *stiffness* in back. As *if it would break.*
• Can't rise up from sitting. Walking impossible.
• Legs give out. Weak, lame, with sensation of HEAVINESS.
• *Full* sensation.
• Left knee stiff and swollen.
• Aching between shoulder blades.

Modalities

< MOTION, WALKING, STOOPING, standing, lying.
< On beginning to move.
< *Rising up from sitting*, right side.
< *Morning*, on waking, during and after sleep.
< During pregnancy or after if menses is delayed or missed.
> HEAT (pain relieved though person is > in *cool* and open air).
> Continued exertion. Kneeling.

AESCULUS HIPPOCASTANUM

▼ SYMPTOM PROFILE

Psychological
- Dull and confused, sluggish on waking. Thinking is an effort.
- Depressed, sad. Very irritable.

Metabolic
- Slow-moving, passive individual.
- Faint, weak, weary. Sense of fullness anywhere in the body.

Veins
- *Hemorrhoids.* Feeling of fullness, heat, burning; as if full of sticks.
- Long-lasting pain, little bleeding < standing, motion, walking.
- Stasis and congestion of the veins and *liver* circulation.

Digestive
- Constipation; hard stool. Fullness of abdomen. Liver congestion.

Gynecological
- Uterine prolapse, pelvic congestion, and "womb consciousness."

▼ DOSAGE

Potency
- Generally low potencies: 3rd to 6th in hemorrhoids.
- Up to the 30th for back pain.

Repetition
- Can be repeated frequently.

▼ CLINICAL CONDITIONS

- Ankylosing spondylitis (early stages)
- Arthritis • Headache • Hemorrhoids
- Low back pain • Sciatica • Sacral pain
- Sacroiliac conditions
- Varicose veins.

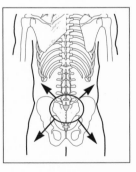

AGARICUS

Fly Agaric

▼ **KEYNOTES**

➤ Back pain with extremely tender, ticklish, or SENSITIVE SPINE.
➤ TWITCHINGS, spasms, incoordination; many *sensory disturbances.*
➤ < Touch, pressure, cold, sitting > Evening, slow motion.

▼ **MUSCULOSKELETAL SYMPTOMS**

Pain
• STITCHING. Like *ice-cold needles.* Tearing, shooting pains.
• Bruised, sprained feeling. Tenderness along the entire spine.

Occiput
• Headache, with stiffness of facial muscles.

Spine
• Like splinters between scapulae. Muscles feel short on bending.
• Feelings of weakness or *coldness* between the shoulder blades.
• Sciatica or LOW BACK PAIN, with radiation into hip joint or legs.
  < Sitting, stooping, standing, MOTION, walking, turning > LYING.
• Pain while lying, yet unable to rise, must lie on the back.
• First and second lumbar vertebrae extremely painful and tender.

Limbs
• Shoulder or hip rheumatism (right side); also wrist, ankle, knees.
• Tearing, drawing, aching pain in buttocks, feet, leg, including sciat-
  ica. < standing, sitting > motion, walking.

Associated
• *Entire spine painful.* Burning pain deep in the spine.
• *Extremely sensitive spine* < touch, leaning against a chair, bathing.
• *Stiffness* of spine. *Cracking,* crepitus of spine.
• Coldness of spine. ICY COLDNESS in spots on the body.
• AWKWARD or uncoordinated movement. *Yawning.*
• TWITCHING, tremors, TREMBLING, spasms, and cramps.
• Creeping, *crawling sensations. Ticklish.* Jerking associated with pains.
• Itching, burning, or cold sensations; tingling or NUMBNESS.
• WEAK muscles, can hardly sit up straight.
• HEAVINESS, tired limbs, both upper and lower extremities.

AGARICUS MUSCARIUS

Modalities
- *Spine:* < MOTION, turning. *Extremities* and trembling > MOTION.
< Pressure on spine. SITTING, STANDING, overexertion. Stooping.
< COLD, open air, *touch, pressure.* Morning, DAYTIME. Right side.
> Gentle motion, walking. *Evening,* sleep.
> *Lying on back.* Lying may either aggravate *or* relieve sacral pain.

▼ Symptom Profile

Psychological
- Opposite or bipolar emotional states. Cheerful, active, and reckless or fearless, followed by lassitude, depression, dullness.
- Weakness of will. Depressed, indifferent, and unable to function or do mental work in the morning > evening.
- Fear of cancer. Nervous and restless.
- Intellectual weakness or exhaustion. Makes many mistakes.
- Mental hyperactivity at night causing insomnia.

Metabolic
- Very CHILLY < cold air. Sweats with the least effort.
- Many sensory and motor disturbances of the nervous system.

▼ Dosage

Potency
- 6the to 30th. In neurological conditions, 30th and higher.

Repetition
- Can be repeated frequently in acute disorders.

▼ Clinical Conditions

Musculoskeletal
- Growing pains • Headache (frontal or temporal) • Low back pain
- Rheumatism • Sciatica • Thoracic pain.

Neurological
- Athetosis • Chorea • Epilepsy • Delirium tremens • Frostbite
- Hyperactivity (in children) • Insomnia • Neuralgia
- Neurological deficit • Tremors, twitches, spasm • Vertigo.

AMMONIUM MUR

NH_4Cl

Ammonium Chloride

▼ KEYNOTES

➣ Subacute or chronic sciatica; shooting into toes with tingling.
➣ CONTRACTURE of muscles, tendons, hamstrings.
➣ < SITTING or walking erect > LYING, walking stooped, warmth.

▼ SCIATICA SYMPTOMS

Pain
- Chronic effects of SPRAINS.
- SHOOTING and TEARING. Vise-like backache. *Contractive* pain.

Location
- Radiating into tips of toes ①. Hips and hamstrings tense.
- Tearing pain from place to place in limbs.

Associated
- CONTRACTION of HAMSTRINGS ②, muscles of hip, knee, foot. < on walking (must walk stooped), but > continued motion.
- TIGHTNESS, tension, *shortening* of muscles, tendons, low back.
- Tingling or formication (crawling sensation) of toe-tips. ③
- Numbness of legs or feet.
- Paralytic weakness and fatigue of legs, *limping*. Walks bent.
- *Pain in heels* ④. Stitches in heels at night in bed > rubbing.
- Foot sweats, though feet are chilly.
- Soreness throughout the body. Bone pains at night.
- Tearing pain in the thighs. Tension in the legs < sitting.
- Pain as if sprained in the groin, prevents standing erect.

Other areas
- *Hips*: Gnawing pains on sitting. Must limp.
- *Knee*: Stitching pain. Swollen, stiff.
- *Thoracic spine*: Shooting pains and *coldness between scapula*.
- *Coccyx* pain on sitting.

Modalities
< SITTING, *walking erect*. Both motion and rest may aggravate.
< Evening, NIGHT, IN BED, during sleep, 3-4 a.m. Open air.

AMMONIUM MURIATICUM

• Sciatica is > LYING, but many pains, tension in legs, and low back pain are < LYING, and < lying on the side or in bed. > WALKING STOOPED. *Warm bath*. CONTINUED MOTION. Rubbing.

▼ SYMPTOM PROFILE

Psychological
• Depression. Suppressed grief, unable to cry. Fear of darkness.
• Hatred towards certain people. Drowsy, unmotivated, sluggish.

Metabolic
• *Chilly*. Feet cold, especially at night. In general < in morning.
• Body large, obese with thin legs. Large buttocks.
• Antidoted by Bitter almonds, Nux vomica, Coffea (the remedy), Causticum.

Respiratory
• Profuse secretions, nasal discharge. Laryngitis. Rattling cough.

Skin
• Itching rashes with eruption of vesicles or pimples.

▼ DOSAGE

Potency
• Generally the 6c, though the 30th or 200th is recommended by some experts.

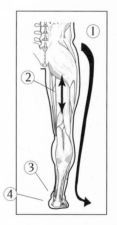

Repetition
• Repeat frequently for pain.
• Once or twice daily in chronic cases.
• Deep-acting enough to result in permanent cure of sciatica.
• A person who needs Ammonium muriaticum should take warm baths, which relieve the symptoms.

▼ CLINICAL CONDITIONS

• Amputation (neuralgia of the stump) • Coccyx pain • Foot pain
• Heel pain • Hemorrhoids • Sciatica • Sprains.

APIS

the Honeybee

▼ KEYNOTES

➤ STINGING and *burning* pain; wandering, migrating.
➤ SWELLING and EDEMA of tissues and around joints.
➤ < HEAT, touch, and pressure > COLD.

▼ MUSCULOSKELETAL SYMPTOMS

Pain
• Stitching, darting, or STINGING pain.
• *Burning*. Sensation like hot needles.
• Sudden onset.

Location
• Serous or synovial membranes, bursa, subcutaneous spaces.
• Pain may *migrate suddenly* from place to place.
• Back, limbs. Affinity to the KNEES, SHOULDERS.
• Knee synovitis with swelling. Swollen feet.

Associated
• EDEMA, SWELLING. Rosy red and inflamed or pink.
• Swollen, shiny, and waxy / transparent.
• AWKWARDNESS, drops things, *clumsy*.
• RESTLESSNESS, fidgety.
• Tired feelings, lassitude with trembling.
• Numbness in upper limbs, hands, or fingertips when grasping.

Modalities
< HEAT in all forms: *local application of heat*.
< Hot or stuffy environment.
< *Touch. Pressure*. Right side or from right to left. Lying.
< Morning. 3-5 p.m. After sleep.
< Exertion, exercise, motion.
> COLD applications, washing. Open air, uncovering.
> SITTING erect. Change of position (causing restlessness).
< Effects of suppressed skin eruptions.

APIS MELLIFICA

▼ **SYMPTOM PROFILE**

Psychological
- BUSY, over-active, or meaningless activity. Business orientation.
- Restless, fidgety, nervous. Lack of perseverance (a busy bee!).
- Childish laughter or silliness.
- JEALOUSY, possessive. Irritable, dictatorial within the family.
- Weeping without cause. Whining.
- Effects of fear, grief, jealousy, rage, shock.

Metabolic
- EDEMA anywhere. Puffy swelling under and around the eyes.
- Debility, prostration; must lie down. Constricted sensations.
- Drowsy but too restless to sleep.

Kidney
- Kidney disease with edema. Nephritis, urinary retention. Cystitis.
- Right-sided ovarian cysts.

Skin
- Urticaria. Hives with burning. Erysipelas. Herpes zoster.

▼ **DOSAGE**

Potency
- 6th to 200th potency (30 for edema).

Repetition
- Can be repeated frequently in low potencies.
- Slow in action. Increased urination may occur during treatment.
- CONTRAINDICATED DURING PREGNANCY.

▼ **CLINICAL CONDITIONS**

- Acute arthritis or rheumatism • Bursitis • Edema • Knee edema (Housemaid's knee) • Rheumatoid arthritis (acute) • Synovitis.

ARGENTUM NIT

AgNO$_3$

Silver Nitrate

▼ KEYNOTES

➤ One-sided or frontal headache. DULL, stupefied, senseless.

➤ *Head feels expanded*, heavy. Chilly, weak, TREMBLING, vomiting.

➤ < Warm room, exertion, stress > Pressure, *bandaging head*, cool air.

▼ HEADACHE SYMPTOMS

Pain

1. Pressing or constriction like a band or loop. Screwing, vise-like.
2. Pulsating 3. Digging, boring, screwing. 4. Stabbing, cutting, or stitching. 5. Tearing. 6. Dull and aching.
• Pains increase gradually and decrease suddenly.

Onset

• On waking. Starts with temporary blindness, sore eyes.

Location

1. ONE-SIDED, temples. 2. Occiput, extending to forehead.
3. Forehead, at the FRONTAL PROMINENCE.

Causes

• *Mental exhaustion* or *overexertion*, overstudy.
• EMOTIONAL upset, *anticipation anxiety*, worry, humiliation.
• GASTRIC causes, after eating or over-eating, cold food, hot coffee.
• Excess sugar • Eyestrain • Physical overexertion, especially *dancing*.

Associated

• Confusion, stupefied. DULLNESS. Incoherence; unable to talk.
• Lies senseless with the eyes closed.
• EXPANDED or enlarged sensation > by bandaging the head.
• HEAVINESS, fullness.
• Itching, crawling of scalp. Hair feels pulled on the vertex.
• COLD, TREMBLING, weakness.
• VERTIGO, tinnitus. Unsteady on the feet. Insomnia, restless sleep.
• *Vomiting of bile* or sour fluid at end of the pain. BELCHING.

Modalities

< WARM ROOM. Stuffy, crowded room. WARM BED. *Left side.*

• •

ARGENTUM NITRICUM

< ON AWAKENING. Menses. Night, drives her out of bed. Sleep.
< Physical or mental exertion. Motion, dancing.
< Emotional stress, excitement. Noise, odors.
> Hard pressure. TIGHT BANDAGING around the head.
> COLD. *Open fresh air*, cold air. After vomiting. Drinking alcohol.
> Bending head backwards. Hot applications.

▼ **SYMPTOM PROFILE**

Psychological
- *Anxiety* neurosis. Performance anxiety regarding exams, failure.
- ANTICIPATION, anxiety & dread before meetings, events, going out.
- *Phobias*: heights, being late, crowds, insanity. *Claustrophobia*.
- Lack of confidence. Desires company. Feels unloved, *forsaken*.
- *Hurried*, IMPULSIVE. Compulsive, obsessive; foolish actions.

Metabolic
- WARM-BLOODED. *Craves fresh air*, wind, cold food, drink or bathing.
- WEAK and TREMBLING.
- Sedentary or business persons.
- Prematurely old-looking, withered, dried up.
- CRAVES SWEETS, which cause diarrhea or headache. Craves salt.

Digestive
- Great FLATULENCE and belching. Gastric ulcer.
- Diarrhea from anxiety or apprehension.

Throat
- Sore throat. Loss of voice or laryngitis in speakers, singers.

▼ **DOSAGE**

Potency
- 6th to 30th or higher.

Repetition
- Repeat when indicated by symptoms.

▼ **CLINICAL CONDITIONS**

- Anxiety • Connective tissue disease • Headache • Migraine
- Parkinson's Disease • Tremors • Tension headache • Vertigo.

ARNICA

Leopard's Bane

▼ KEYNOTES

➣ TRAUMA: First remedy for injury, bruising, etc. Fear after injury.
➣ Muscular strain or fatigue. Restless. Mental & physical SHOCK.
➣ Sore, bruised pain < LEAST TOUCH, jarring, at night.

▼ MUSCULOSKELETAL SYMPTOMS

Pain
• SORE, *bruised*, beaten sensation of the part, or of the whole body.
• Hypersensitive to pain. Pain of parts lain on.

Associated
• RESTLESS; no comfortable place; bed feels too hard.
• EXHAUSTION and *weakness* after exertion or trauma.
• Face and head are hot — body and nose are cold.
• Cold extremities, with feeling of internal heat (effects of shock).

Modalities
< TOUCH or contact. *Jarring*, sudden motions or exertion.
< At rest. Lying on one side or area too long. At *night*, after sleep.
< *Damp, cold*, from becoming overheated.
< After wine (has an adverse effect on those requiring Arnica).
> COLD applications. Open air. Changing position.
> Lying down or *with the head low*. Sitting erect. Lying outstretched.

Psychological
• FEAR after accidents < night, when alone. *Worry over small ailments.*
• *Fear of touch* or approach of anyone. Fear of death, disease, crowds.
• *Insomnia*, starting from sleep; *nightmares after injury*, dreams of accidents.
• SHOCK after injury. Hyposensitive: delirium or stupor.
• Feels nothing is wrong, sends the doctor away. Wants solitude.
• IRRITABLE, oversensitive; averse to sympathy. Silent.

▼ EXTERNAL USE

• Bruises or "charley horse," muscular strains or overexertion.
• Strengthens the hair and scalp.
• Not for use where the skin is broken i.e., open wounds or scrapes.

8 •

ARNICA MONTANA

▼ DOSAGE

Potency

- For recent conditions: 6, 12, or 30, though one can use high potencies successfully in cases of acute trauma (200, 1M).
- In conditions stemming from injury in the past ("never well since"), single or weekly doses of the 200, 1M, or 10M are very effective.
- Externally, use homeopathic (from live plants) tincture (1x or ø).

Repetition

- Repeat frequently for acute; from every five minutes to hourly.
- Reduce dosage over several days with improvement.
- Three times daily for long-term use or recuperation.

▼ CLINICAL CONDITIONS

- TRAUMA: Falls, sprains, blows, wounds, fracture; soft tissue injury.
  — Reduces and prevents pain, bleeding, bruising, swelling.
  — Prevents secondary infection, accelerates healing.
- BRUISING: Reduces or prevents bruising, bleeding, hematoma.
- SHOCK: Mental and physical shock from injury, loss, grief.
- *Past injury*: For the after-effects of trauma in the remote past. Never well or recovered since an injury, fall, or trauma.
- MUSCULAR strains, sprains, bruising or "charley horse."
- *Overexertion*: Of muscles, cardiovascular (athlete's heart), voice.
- *Exercise*: Relaxes muscle tone, improves stamina, reduces injury.
- *Surgery*: Before and after operations, dental work, post-partum.
- *Manipulation*: Use before or after joint manipulation.
- *Preventive*: Useful before exercise, surgery, or unusual exertion.
- ENT: Eye injuries (prevents traumatic cataract), loss of vision after injury, retinal hemorrhage; blows to the ear, nosebleeds.
- *Head*: Head injury or concussion (see Hypericum).
- *Stroke*: Both in acute stages and for assisting recovery.
- *Insomnia*: From overexertion, injuries, accidents, with nightmares.
- *Rheumatism* or gout, with fear of touch.
- *Spine*: Neck & low back pain; soreness with stitching, tenderness.

ARSENICUM

As$_2$O$_3$

Oxide of Arsenic

▼ KEYNOTES

➤ BURNING, shooting, tearing pain, with CHILLINESS.
➤ ANXIETY, RESTLESSNESS, and WEAKNESS. Trembling.
➤ < Cold, NIGHT, violent exertion > HEAT, walking, gentle motion.

▼ SCIATICA SYMPTOMS

Pain

- Intermittent sudden attacks of pain < at night with anxiety, chilliness, weakness, and need to lie down.
- BURNING, like fire, like hot needles. Boiling sensation.
- Tearing, sharp, drawing, or shooting. Unbearably intense.
- Sciatica from COLD or working in cold, damp places.

Location

- From HIP, to thighs, legs, calf, heels or down to tips of toes.
- Limbs and feet weary, WEAK, numb, and swollen.
- Knee pains, as if beaten.
- Cramps in calves. Must keep legs and feet in motion.
- Brachial neuralgia with tearing pain from elbows to shoulder.
- *Low back*: as if broken, burning pain. Pain in sacrum or coccyx.

Associated

- RESTLESSNESS in general and in limbs and feet. Must move.
- WEAKNESS, debility. *Exhaustion*. Loss of strength.
- Trembling, twitching, spasm, tingling and heaviness in limbs.
- CHILLY; coldness of extremities; Raynaud's syndrome.
- ANXIETY, nervousness.
- Paralysis and atrophy.
- Swelling, EDEMA. Puffiness in extremities.

Modalities

< NIGHT, after midnight. COLD (except headache). DAMP.
< Vigorous motion or *exertion*. Ascending.
< *Right side*. Lying on affected side, with the head low.

9

ARSENICUM ALBUM

> WARMTH in all forms. Hot *applications*. Sweating. Keeping busy.
> WALKING, moving about, gentle motion. Flexing the limbs.
> Lying with head elevated. Descending.

▼ SYMPTOM PROFILE

Psychological
- Insecurity, ANXIETY, fear of death, of being alone, about health.
- SUSPICIOUS, controlled, tight. Critical or vindictive.
- Proper, *perfectionist*, FASTIDIOUS. Demanding and controlling.
- Chronic depression with *despair of recovery*; suicidal. Selfish.
- Greedy, miserly, possessive; hoarding or collecting.

Metabolic
- CHILLY. Nervous and RESTLESS.
- *Periodicity*: Recurrent or cyclic conditions; daily, weekly, monthly, annually. At the same time daily.
- EXHAUSTION from the slightest exertion; low vitality.

Head
- Dull heavy pain in forehead, occiput, root of nose.

Digestive
- Diarrheas and dysentery, colitis. Food poisoning, gastritis.

Respiratory
- Colds, influenza, hay fever. Asthma < midnight. Emphysema.

▼ DOSAGE

Potency
- Effective in all potencies. Low potencies for local conditions.
- High for neurological, psychological, or constitutional symptoms.

Repetition
- Frequent repetitions may be used in acute conditions.
- In chronic conditions, a single dose and wait until indicated again.

▼ CLINICAL CONDITIONS

- Brachial neuralgia • Coccyx pain • Low back pain • Neuralgia
- Neuritis • Raynaud's syndrome • Rheumatism • Sacral pain
- Sciatica.

BELLADONNA

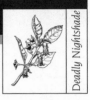

Deadly Nightshade

▼ KEYNOTES

➢ Headache with intense, sudden onset, heat & flushing. *Throbbing*.
➢ Acute inflammation of joints: swelling, redness, spasm.
➢ < Motion, stooping, drafts, light, noise, jarring > LYING, warmth.

▼ HEADACHE SYMPTOMS

Pain
- *Sudden*, VIOLENT, intense onset of vascular congestion.
- Start and cease very suddenly, but last indefinitely.
- *Throbbing*, pulsating. Stabbing like a knife, burning.
- PRESSURE in forehead, pressing in or out, as if bursting.
- Shocks, bangs, jerking or wavy sensations inside the head.
- *Causes*: Suppressed nasal discharge, fever, colds or chill, after a haircut or putting the hair up, concussion, sun exposure, migraine.

Location
- FOREHEAD (temples, occiput) or unilateral (right).

Associated
- Hot, flushed, restless, and congested. Dilated pupils. HOT HEAD with cold hands and feet. Hypersensitivity of all senses. RESTLESS.
- *Bores head into pillow*. Sensitive scalp. Cannot open eyes from pain.
- Dry mouth, nose, tongue. *Nosebleeds* with headache.
- Bounding pulse. Throbbing of carotid arteries. Vertigo.
- Jerking, falling, wobbling or shaking of head. Sensation of sinking and rising. HEAVINESS, fullness of the head.

▼ MUSCULOSKELETAL SYMPTOMS

- *Joints*: Heat, redness, throbbing, sensitive to touch. Acute arthritis or rheumatism with headache, fever, throbbing pulse. *Iritis*.
- *Spine*: Burning, throbbing. Gnawing and shooting pain in spinal column. Arthritic pain *as if it would break*, pain from within outward.
- *Neck*: Stiff, swollen < bending head back, touch. Tearing, cutting pain in shoulder, shooting down arm.
- *Low Back and Sciatica*: Cramp-like pain and soreness in lumbar spine,

10

ATROPA BELLADONNA

coccyx < touch > standing upright (sometimes <), walking.
- Acute curvature of low back (from spasm). Bearing down in sacrum.
- *Knee & hip*: Pain < sitting > standing, walking.

Modalities
< Light, noise, SUN, cold or open air, drafts. Walking in the wind, getting wet. Afternoon and NIGHT.
< MOTION, least exertion, moving the eyes, bending head forward, right side. Rising from sitting. STOOPING. *Jarring* or misstep.
> LYING (headache), in a dark room. Bending head backwards.
> Warm wraps or warm room, standing. Closing the eyes. Pressure.
> Leaning on something, lying on painful side with head high.

▼ SYMPTOM PROFILE

Psychological
- FEARFUL, desire to run away, excitable, VIOLENT. Delirium, wild imaginings OR withdrawn, dull, confused. Moaning. *Agonizing pain.*

Metabolic
- Acute infections, first stages of inflammation anywhere in the body. Flashes or rushes of blood to the head and various areas.

▼ DOSAGE

Potency
- Use the 6, 12, or 30 in inflammatory and spasmodic conditions, higher potencies if mental and keynote symptoms are present.

Repetition
- Hourly doses in acute cases, until improvement.
- In subacute cases, three times daily or as symptoms require.

▼ CLINICAL CONDITIONS

Musculoskeletal: • Acute joint inflammation: bursitis, synovitis, arthritis • Headache • Low back pain • Sciatica.
Other Systems: • Acute fevers • Appendicitis • Bronchitis • Conjunctivitis • Cystitis • Gastric spasm • Laryngitis • Mastitis • Otitis media • Peritonitis. • Strep throat or scarlet fever • Tonsillitis.

BELLIS

Common Daisy

▼ KEYNOTES

➤ Trauma: like Arnica but for deeper tissues. Intense SORENESS.

➤ REPETITIVE STRAIN, sprains. Swelling and bruising.

➤ < TOUCH, Chilling > Motion, rubbing. Intense fatigue.

▼ MUSCULOSKELETAL SYMPTOMS

Pain
• Intense SORENESS all over; bruised, aching sensation.

Location
• Muscles, soft tissue, abdomen, pelvis, breasts, legs, wrists.

Associated
• SWELLING from injuries, especially where Arnica fails to relieve.
• BRUISING, contusions; sensitive to the touch (< lower limbs).
• *Coldness* of injured limb or area.

Causes and Conditions
• INJURY: like Arnica, but deeper trauma, more *swelling and bruising.*
• MUSCULAR fatigue or overstrain; *prolonged standing.*
• Effects of falls, injuries, blows, sprains in the REMOTE PAST.
• Effects of REPETITIVE STRAIN, manual labor, microtrauma result-
ing in arthritis or rheumatism. Contractive pain in wrist.
• OLD BACK STRAINS. Injuries to the coccyx.
• Trauma to abdomen, pelvic organs, or lower limbs.
• *After surgery* (main remedy). Surgical trauma; pain and bruising.
• GETTING CHILLED after overheating or after a cold bath.
• Prolonged travel, jostling, jarring (motorcycles, pneumatic drills).
• *Wrist:* as if bandaged. Dislocated. Tendon contraction.
• Tumors at the site of an old injury.
• PREGNANCY: Back strain or sore abdomen from fetal movement.

Modalities
< Getting CHILLED when hot. Cold drinks when overheated.
< Getting wet, cold bath, or drinks. Before a storm.
< TOUCH. Warmth of bed, hot bathing. Left side.
> Continued motion. Rubbing. Rest, lying down. Cold locally.

11

BELLIS PERENNIS

▼ SYMPTOM PROFILE

Metabolic
- *Exhausted*, intense fatigue and *wish to lie down*.
- Wakes at 3 a.m. or wakes early and cannot get back to sleep.

Stomach
- Indigestion or stomach ache, vomiting, or regurgitation.
- < Cold drinks, when overheated, touch.
- Pain > eating and pressure.
- Spleen disorders.

Female Conditions
- Backache or strain during pregnancy.
- Uterine strain, soreness; from prolonged standing or pregnancy.
- Varicose veins during pregnancy.
- BREAST inflammation or tumor at the site of an INJURY or bruise.

Skin
- Acne, boils, and abscess. Bruising. Varicose veins.

▼ DOSAGE

Potency
- Low potencies: 3, 6, 12, or 30.
- Tincture (Ø) applied externally to sore areas or breast tissue.

Repetition
- *Acute*: Frequent repetition (hourly) in acute conditions or trauma.
- *Chronic*: Three times daily in chronic conditions.
  Note: Do not use too close to bed time, as it may cause insomnia.

▼ CLINICAL CONDITIONS

- Bruises • Carpal tunnel syndrome • Gout • Old injuries
- Repetitive strain • Rheumatism • Swelling • Trauma.

BERBERIS

Barberry

▼ KEYNOTES

➤ Stitching, tearing low back pain, RADIATING in any direction.
➤ < MOTION, rising from sitting, standing, lying. Numb, stiff, lame.
➤ Weakness of lower limbs. Kidney or liver symptoms.

▼ LOW BACK SYMPTOMS

Pain
- Sharp, stitching, TEARING, bruised sensation in the back, neck.
- Sudden twinges of pain. *Rapidly changing pains and location.*

Location
- *Low back*: One-sided pain, upper lumbar, or entire lumbar spine.
- Kidney area. Sacral pain.
- RADIATING in all directions:
    — outward, up or down from the low back area.
    — to the whole body.
    — to the abdomen, groin, pelvis, hips, buttock, or back of thighs.
    — down the *front of thighs* to the legs or calves.
- *Foot pain*: Burning, cutting pain on stepping or standing on balls of feet, though weight on the heels is okay. Pain in soles like a nail.
- *Knee*: Left knee painful, lame < rising from a seat. SWOLLEN, stiff.

Associated
- NUMBNESS, *stiffness*, WEAKNESS. As if paralyzed.
- Lower limbs *weak, lame* < after walking. Can barely walk.
- *Rise from sitting* is painful and difficult. Has to support the back.
- Kidney area *tender* with burning, soreness.
- Bubbling, boiling, gurgling, water-like sensations.
- Heat or warmth in lumbar spine.
- Tension in the sacrum.

Modalities
< MOTION, *jarring*, jumping or stepping hard, walking.
< *Rising from a seat.*
< Standing. LYING (especially in A.M.). Stooping. Sitting.

BERBERIS VULGARIS

< Right or left side.
< With fatigue. May or may not be < pressure.
< Morning, on waking. During menses.
> Afternoon.

▼ Symptom Profile

Psychological
- *Indifferent*, apathetic, desires company. Concentration difficult.
- Anxiety at twilight, fear of darkness.

Metabolic
- Weakness, lassitude. Faintness. Greyish complexion. Dry mouth.
- Dark circles around eyes. As if a tight cap around head.

Genitourinary
- Urging and burning with pain extending to lumbar spine, hips, legs. Red sediment in urine. Dysmenorrhea with radiating pains.
- Renal colic. Kidney stones. Cystitis.

Liver/Gall Bladder
- Gallstones, gall bladder colic with pain in left shoulder. Jaundice.

▼ Dosage

Potency
- 6, 12, or 30 for local illness.
- 200 if characteristic symptoms are present.

Repetition
- Three times daily or more in acute phases or for local treatment of organ.
- Single dose of higher potencies.

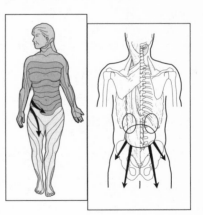

▼ Clinical Conditions

- Foot disorders • Gout • Knee bursitis • Low back pain
- Lumbar neuralgia • Rheumatism • Sciatica • Shoulder bursitis.

BRYONIA

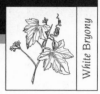

White Bryony

▼ KEYNOTES

➤ *Inflammation* of joints & bursa with *stitching* pains. IRRITABILITY.
➤ Migraine; bursting, hammering, with red face, hot head.
➤ < MOTION, stooping, touch, hot room > REST, *pressure*, local heat.

▼ MUSCULOSKELETAL SYMPTOMS

• STITCHING, sharp, cutting. *Tearing*, drawing.
• Onset can be gradual (arthritis) or sudden (injuries or fracture).
• *Neck*: Stiffness, tension in nape.
• *Thorax*: Stitches from scapulae and spine through to heart.
• *Low Back*: Tearing, drawing pains in lumbar and sacral spine
  < bending, sitting up, turning. As if beaten. *Must walk or sit bent over.*

Associated

• HOT, RED, SWOLLEN and shiny, or pale red and puffy.
• Lies or sits perfectly still, dreading any motion whatsoever.
• *Irritability*. Sore and sensitive to touch.
• *Constipation*: hard, dry stools. Heartburn, *indigestion*, heaviness.

Modalities

< SLIGHTEST MOTION: S*tooping*, exertion, *jarring*, rising up, turning,
  walking, stretching, raising the leg, coughing, deep breath, sneezing, straining, motion of the head, eyes, ascending, rising up.
< TOUCH. Eating. When constipated. Left side.
< *Becoming* HOT or hot room, from cold weather to warm. Chilling.
< In cold, wet weather, cold wind, COLD BATHING, weather changes.
< MORNING, on waking; 3 a.m. or 9 p.m. (late evening).
> IMMOBILIZATION: Lying or *lying on painful side* (except headache).
> PRESSURE, tight bandaging, bracing the area. REST, quiet.
> Heat *to inflamed areas*, though better cool in general. Perspiring.
> Cool open air. Overcast or damp weather. Closing eyes.

Psychological

• IRRITABILITY and anger < if disturbed. Seeks quiet and solitude.
• *Worries about business*. Fear of poverty, the future, change.

13

BRYONIA ALBA

▼ **HEADACHE SYMPTOMS**
- *Starts in morning* on first moving eyes. Gradually increases till p.m.
- BURSTING, SPLITTING, sharp, *stitching*. Hammering inside.
- HEAVY HEAD. Crushing weight. *Pressing in or bursting out.*
- Back of head (occiput), FRONTAL, into cheeks or eye. Right or left.
- Spreads to the whole body from the occiput or temples.
- On stooping, feels as if contents of head would come out.
- *Causes*: Anger, fright, contradiction, overeating, constipation, liver congestion, cold air, chilling, cold drinks when overheated, coffee.

Modalities as before, plus the following:
- < Stooping, coughing, after eating, light, noise, motion of eyes. SUN.
- > Lying with the head low, WRAPPING UP HEAD. *Closing the eyes.*
- > HEAT or warm applications (though head is HOT).
- Temple pain < lying on it. Occiput pain > lying on it.

Associated
- *Thirst* for large quantities. *Dryness* of lips, mouth, throat.
- White or yellow coated tongue, *bitter taste*. Constipation or diarrhea.
- Vertigo: Dizzy or faint on rising.
- Head HOT, *red face*, but body cold. Nosebleeds, *rushes of blood to head*.
- Scalp sore and sensitive.

▼ **DOSAGE**
Potency
- 6, 12, or 30. Low potencies in gout, rheumatism, inflammation.

Repetition
- Short-acting, Bryonia bears frequent repetition during acute stages or symptoms. Otherwise, one to three times daily.

▼ **CLINICAL CONDITIONS**

- Arthritis (acute) • Bursitis • Dislocations • Fibrositis, fibromyalgia
- Fractures (pain) • Knee synovitis • Low back pain • Migraine (acute)
- Myalgia • Myositis • Rheumatoid conditions • Sciatica
- Sprains • Strains • Subluxations • Synovitis • Tendonitis
- Tension headache • Torticollis • Trauma (if Arnica fails to help).

CALC CARB

$CaCO_3$

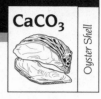

Oyster Shell

▼ **KEYNOTES**

➤ Arthritis, chronic strains, effects of overlifting. Follows Rhus tox.
➤ "As if sprained." Stiffness. Nodosities. Spinal pain, curvature.
➤ < Cold, damp, motion or overexertion > Lying, standing, warmth.

▼ **MUSCULOSKELETAL SYMPTOMS**

Pain & Associated Symptoms

• Sprained sensation. Varied pains: cutting, shooting, tearing.
• *Nodosities* of the shoulder, wrist, hands, fingers.
• *Contraction* of muscles and tendons of hand, fingers, knee, ankle.
• STIFFNESS. Weakness or lameness of joints. Muscular weakness.
• Effects of chronic or recurrent sprains. Easy overstraining.
• Numbness of side lain on. Lump sensation in neck or thorax.

Locations

• SPINE: *Weakness of back*; difficult to sit upright. Curvatures.
  Osteophytes, spinal arthritis. Vertebrae feel loose. Painful stiffness.
  Painful or tender vertebrae (especially neck, thorax). Stitching pain.
• NECK: *Stiff*, rigid at base of neck, from overlifting, with headache.
  Tension and pain prevent turning. Stitches while talking. Thin or
  scrawny neck. Cramping pain extending to vertex. Swelling at C7.
  Burning in base of neck and occiput, all day but > going to sleep.
• THORAX: Pressure, drawing pain between or under shoulder
  blades, impeding breathing < inspiration, motion. Shooting pain
  extends to arms < motion > standing. Sudden stitches.
  Curvature of thoracic spine. Itching, numbness, or lump sensation.
• LOW BACK: Pain from overlifting, feels as if sprained. Can't rise
  from seat due to pain. < night, jarring. Weakness. Rheumatism.
• *Sacrum* and *Coccyx*: Heat in tailbone. Drawing and pinching pains.
• *Shoulder* rheumatism, brachial neuralgia with weak, lame arms.
• *Hands*: Arthritis of hands, fingers. Nodosities. Cramps, atrophy.
• *Hips*: Arthritis with contraction, cutting, shooting pain. Dislocation.
• *Knees*: SWOLLEN, hot, red, with stitching, tearing pains. *Weak knees*.
• Cramps in calf, hollow of knee, soles of feet. Heavy, tired limbs.

14

• •

CALCAREA CARBONICA

• *Feet*: Weak ankles, pain in Achilles tendon. Cramps in soles of feet.

Modalities

< COLD, DAMP, getting wet. Night (pain). Morning (stiffness).

< MOTION, over-exertion, bending back, turning, straightening the spine, stretching, deep breath, sitting, rising up. Rest.

> Standing. Warmth, dry weather. Rubbing.

> LYING, *lying on back* or lying on the painful side. Lying on abdomen.

▼ SYMPTOM PROFILE

Psychological

• Conscientious, RESPONSIBLE. Hard-working but unimaginative.

• FEARS and insecurity. Phobias of insects, mice. Anxiety regarding health, insanity, poverty, being observed.

Metabolic

• Obese, fleshy, pale, lack of muscular tone, flabby. Oyster-like!

• WEAKNESS. Lack of endurance, resilience, or stamina.

• CHILLY. *Cold, clammy* feet and hands. At night, feet freezing at first, then get overheated.

• Profuse *sour perspiration*; from exertion, at night, from the cold.

• Glandular swelling: in and around neck, margins of hair.

▼ DOSAGE

Potency

• 6th to 30th. High potencies if constitutional symptoms match.

Repetition

• Daily repetition of lower potencies or single dose of high.

▼ CLINICAL CONDITIONS

• Arthritis (osteoarthritis, rheumatoid or psoriatic arthritis) • Brachial neuralgia • Chronic sprains • Coccyx (tailbone) pain • Connective tissue disease • Dislocations • Fibrositis • Gout • Headache • Hip joint disease • Kyphosis • Low back pain • Lupus • Nodosities • Osteomalacia (Rickets) • Osteoporosis • Rheumatism • Sciatica • Scoliosis • Spina bifida • Spondylosis • Tennis elbow • Torticollis• Trauma (overlifting) • Wrist ganglion.

CALC FLUOR

CaF_2

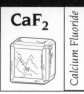

Calcium Fluoride

▼ KEYNOTES

➤ WEAK, stretched ligaments, chronic strains. ADHESIONS.

➤ HARDENING around joints; nodules, deposits. Stiffness.

➤ Chronic cases where Rhus tox is indicated but fails to work.

▼ MUSCULOSKELETAL SYMPTOMS

Pain

• Burning pain. Grinding, sharp, darting pains.

• Chronic cases with Rhus tox type of symptoms.

Joints

• WEAK LIGAMENTS; easy strains or dislocations.

• Chronic and recurrent sprains, overexertion resulting in stretched ligaments or in arthritic joints and deposits.

• Laborers, athletes or dancers who overstrain joints, muscles.

• Joint "mice" — fragments or deposits of bone or cartilage in the joints (knee, wrist, ankles, etc). Bony growths at site of an injury.

• *Fibrous nodules*, enlargements in tendons, ligaments, joints.

Locations

• LOW BACK PAIN < after rest > moving, warmth. Weak, dragging, bearing down pain. Fullness, burning. After strain. *Chronic*. Tired, aching, even after sitting a short time.

• NECK PAIN < cold and drafts > heat.

• HIP joint disease. Spontaneous dislocation.

• KNEE synovitis, swelling, bursitis (Housemaid's knee), cysts. Trembling of knees from weakness. Cramp in calves at night.

• WRIST: Ganglion, tumors, cysts.

• HANDS: Arthritis nodosities, exostoses of fingers. Dupuytren's contracture. Burning of palms and soles.

Associated

• STIFFNESS of joints.

• RESTLESSNESS with backache.

• CRACKING and creaking of joints. Lack of lubrication.

15

CALCAREA FLUORICA

Modalities

< BEGINNING MOTION, *after rest*. Sitting. On waking.
< COLD, *damp*, weather changes. Drafts.
> *Continued motion* (limbering up), walking about, stretching.
> WARM APPLICATIONS, heat. Rubbing.

▼ **SYMPTOM PROFILE**

Psychological

• Fear of poverty, of FINANCIAL RUIN (though unjustified).
• Instability, makes many mistakes. Irregular or ineffectual actions.
• Vivid dreams of new places, of effort and striving, of death.

Metabolic

• Fatigue. CHILLY.
• Asymmetrical or anomalous features or anatomy.
• CLUMSY, uncoordinated movements. "Double jointed."
• SCLEROSIS: Used in conditions where there is *hardening of tissue* including hard, swollen lymph nodes, varicose veins, enlarged prostate, goiter, bone tumors, calluses, etc. Aortic aneurysm.
• WEAKNESS of connective tissue: Tooth decay, uterine prolapse.
• ADHESIONS, scars, keloids, with white skin, itching, hard tissue.

▼ **DOSAGE**

Potency

• Lower potencies for bone and joint problems.
• Higher potencies for constitutional or characteristic indications.

Repetition

• Frequent repetitions (once or twice daily) in low potency.

▼ **CLINICAL CONDITIONS**

• Arthritis • Baker's cyst (chronic) • Bone spurs • Bone tumors, cysts
• Bursitis, synovitis (chronic) • Exostoses • Gout • Hip joint disease
• Joint deposits • Knee conditions (chronic) • Low back pain
• Nodules in ligaments, muscles, tendons • Osteophytosis
• *Scar tissue* and adhesions (actual scars or prevention after surgery)
• Sciatica • Scoliosis • Sprains (chronic) • Wrist ganglion.

CALC PHOS

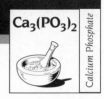

$Ca_3(PO_3)_2$

Calcium Phosphate

▼ KEYNOTES

➢ Rheumatism, arthritis. Stiffness, nodosities, contracture, cramps.
➢ Pains shooting, as if dislocated. Bone disease, weakness.
➢ < COLD, WET, DRAFTS, motion, exertion > Lying, dry weather.

▼ MUSCULOSKELETAL SYMPTOMS

Pain

• *Pain in small spots.* SHOOTING, flies in all directions. Changing locations. "As if beaten." Aching in limbs with weariness.
• Rheumatic inflammation, pain in all joints. EXTENSORS affected more than flexors. Lame flexors, aching extensors.

Locations

• Right, then left side.
• SPINE: Scoliosis with curvature to the left. Spina bifida. Weakness.
• NECK: Weak, thin, heavy. Pain, *stiffness* < slightest draft of air, with dullness in head. Cramping pain alternating one side to the other.
• THORAX: Pain around and below shoulder blades.
• LOW BACK: Violent pain < least effort. Screams with pain < lifting, sneezing. Crick in the back.
• SACROILIAC: Soreness, tearing, shooting. Stitching in left SI joint. Pain as if dislocated or broken < walking. *Sacrum* feels numb, lame.
• COCCYX: Aching, sore, stitching or shooting pains.
• SHOULDER: Aching, tearing in shoulder and shooting down arm.
• ARM: Pain from collarbone to wrist. Aching of whole arm, into thumb. Cannot lift arm. *Trembling.* Elbow pain on right, then left.
• WRIST: Burning, cramping, as if beaten. Lameness < motion.
• HIP disease. Buttocks go to sleep, stinging painful spots. Shooting in thighs, as if beaten, pain in tendons of inner thigh. Weak hip.
• LEGS: Restless, crawling, tingling, lame, heavy. CRAMPS in calves.
• KNEE: Swelling, pain from left to right. Sore < stretching, walking.
• ANKLE: Cramp-like pain, as if dislocated. Aching heels.
• HEADACHE: Of students with anemia and depression, from overwork, *from the neck.* Pain along sutures > cool bathing.

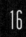

16

• •

CALCAREA PHOSPHORICA

Associated
• WEAK JOINTS. Rheumatism after every cold. After getting wet.
• Limbs (arms, hands, legs) *fall asleep easily*. Chills or heat in spine.
• STIFFNESS < after rest, morning. Contracture, deformity of joints.

Modalities
< DRAFTS, cold wind. COLD DAMP or COLD AIR. Snow air. Weather changes. Getting wet or soaked. Before or during menses.
< Onset in autumn < in winter > in spring.
< MOTION, exertion. LIFTING. Bending back.
Warm, dry. LYING.

▼ SYMPTOM PROFILE

Psychological
• Exhausted by mental work. Complaining, sensitive.
• Indifference, loss of motivation. *Sighing with joint complaints.*
• DISCONTENT, dissatisfaction, boredom. Desire for travel, change.

Metabolic
• *Chilliness.* Cold hands, legs, *buttocks*.
• Delayed development in walking, dentition, closure of fontanelles.
• WEAKNESS and WEARINESS. Emaciation.

▼ DOSAGE

Potency
• 3x to 200. Low potency contraindicated in elderly people.

Repetition
• Can be repeated frequently in low potencies or acute states.

▼ CLINICAL CONDITIONS

• Arthritis • Bone deformity • Brachial neuralgia (Arm pain)
• Carpal tunnel syndrome • Cervical pain • Coccyx pain
• Fracture (non-union or delayed union) • Growing pains • Headache
• Hip joint disease • Leg cramps • Low back pain • Nodosities (gout, arthritis) • Osteomalacia or rickets) • Osteophytes • Osteoporosis
• Restless leg syndrome • Rheumatism • Sacroiliac strain, arthritis
• Sciatica • Scoliosis • Shoulder, hand, arm syndrome • Spina bifida
• Spinal injury (from lifting) • Tendonitis • Tennis elbow • Torticollis.

CALENDULA

Marigold

▼ KEYNOTES

➤ TRAUMA: External treatment of wounds, cuts, abrasions, burns.
➤ Skin infection, irritation, itching, chapping.
➤ Antiseptic and healing for all skin diseases, eyes, mouth.

▼ MUSCULOSKELETAL SYMPTOMS

Trauma

• WOUNDS, cuts, abrasions, lacerations, broken skin surface.
• Rapid healing of wounds, actually sealing the edges and promoting healing by first intention: prevents scar tissue formation.
• Arrests BLEEDING from wounds, especially to scalp, mouth.
• BURNS: scalds, sunburn. Rapidly soothes pain and speeds healing.
• ANTISEPTIC: sores, abscesses, infection at the site of a wound. Both prevents and heals infection, pus formation.
• Wounds are raw, inflamed; red around the edges.
• PAIN out of proportion to actual injury. Painful as if beaten. Pain appears or is *worse after bandage is put on*.
• Exhaustion from blood loss or pain.
• MUSCLE injury: rupture of muscles, tendon.
• FRACTURES or compound fracture. Head injury or concussion.
• Penetrating wounds into joints. Dislocation with soft tissue injury.

Modalities

< *Damp*, CLOUDY weather, open air. Evening.
< Touch, pressure.
> Warmth. Walking. Lying still.

▼ SYMPTOM PROFILE

Psychological

• Nervous and restless. ANXIETY, fear that something will happen.

Metabolic

• Take cold easily in damp weather.
• COLD, sensitive to open air. Restless at night.

CALENDULA OFFICINALIS

▼ CLINICAL CONDITIONS

Skin
- Non-suppressive external treatment of eczema, psoriasis, rashes, dermatitis, itching, irritations, chapping, cracking, etc.
- Topical treatment of fissures, varicose ulcers, bedsores, gangrene.
- Skin infections, including erysipelas • Neuroma • Ulcers.

Eye
- Eyewash for irritations, abrasions, infections, conjunctivitis, eye inflammation after trauma. Wounds to the lids or brows.

Mouth: Mouthwash for bleeding gums, sores, ulcers, surgery.

Ear: Deafness < dampness or with eczema.

Digestive
- Heartburn and nausea with goose flesh. Distention.
- Nausea felt in the chest • Liver remedy: jaundice.

Women
- Cervicitis, HPV, cervical dysplasia (e.g. genital warts). *Cancer remedy.*

Joints
- Rheumatism, drawing pain, only during motion.

▼ DOSAGE

Potency
- TINCTURE: A 10% alcohol solution that should be diluted 1/2 teaspoon per cup of water, or 1:5 for application to cuts, wounds, burns, and *moist* skin conditions, such as eczema or infections.
- LOTION, CREAM, or GEL: In a base of lanolin, Vaseline, or oil. For *dry*, chapped, or cracked skin disorders, such as psoriasis.
- SUCCUS: A pressed extract of Calendula flowers with less alcohol.
- Internal Use: Can be used in potency, up to the 30th.

Repetition
- Can be applied several times daily as a wash or gel, or kept on an area as a moist compress. Internally, use once or more daily.

CAULOPHYLLUM

Blue Cohosh

▼ KEYNOTES

➤ Arthritis of the SMALL JOINTS: hands, feet, neck, low back.
➤ Wandering, cutting or drawing pains. STIFFNESS, nodosities.
➤ GYNECOLOGICAL disturbances. NERVOUS. Weakness, trembling.

▼ MUSCULOSKELETAL SYMPTOMS

Pain
• WANDERING, erratic, or shooting pains (in the limbs), changing place every few minutes.
• *Drawing* or *cutting* pains. Aching, soreness in joints.
• Pain in hands or fingers, felt on closing the hands or grasping.

Location
• SMALL JOINTS, particularly of the hands (but also feet), fingers, toes, wrist, ankles, elbow, or arthritis only of the hands.
• *Spine*: Aching soreness, as if beaten. Headache arising from neck.
• *Neck*: Pains in extremities eventually settle in the nape of the neck. Neck stiffness; drawn to the left side.
• *Low back pain* before menses > during menses.
• *Lower limbs* aching and sore. Hip joint disease.

Associated
• STIFFNESS. Nodosities or joint deposits, exostoses.
• Cracking of joints.
• Restless at night due to pain.
• Swelling and inflammation of the fingers.
• Various GYNECOLOGICAL disturbances; menopause, pregnancy.

Modalities
Arthritis < before menses and > during the flow.
< Clenching hands or gripping. Open air. *Coffee*. Evening.
> Warmth, warm clothing. After menses.

18

CAULOPHYLLUM THALICTROIDES

▼ SYMPTOM PROFILE

Psychological
- NERVOUS, excitable, restless state.
- *Hysteria*; changeable moods. Irritable.
- Anxiety and fears. All mental symptoms < menses.

Metabolic
- Largely a woman's remedy. Rheumatism accompanying gynecological conditions or menstrual/hormonal disturbances.
- WEAKNESS and exhaustion.
- CHILLY. *Internal trembling.*

Face
- Brown spots on the forehead. Weak and drooping eyelids.

Female
- Spasmodic dysmenorrhea; shooting, wandering pains.
- Menopause, prevention of miscarriage, delayed labor, during pregnancy, vaginitis. Uterine atony; prolapse or displacements.

Digestive
- Spasms of stomach (cardialgia). Dyspepsia.

▼ DOSAGE

Potency
- Low potencies: 3, 6, 12, or 30 in joint problems.

Repetition
- Can be repeated several times daily for several weeks.

▼ CLINICAL CONDITIONS

- Arthritis (of small joints) • Arthritis deformans or nodosities of the fingers and hands • Hallux valgus • Hip joint disease
- Low back pain • Neck pain • Torticollis.

CAUSTICUM

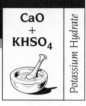

CaO
+
KHSO₄

Potassium Hydrate

▼ KEYNOTES

➤ CONTRACTION, stiffness of tendons, muscles. Joint deformity.
➤ Restlessness < at night. Progressive weakness. Paralysis.
➤ < COLD, dry, evening > Warmth, warm bed, wet, rainy weather.

▼ MUSCULOSKELETAL SYMPTOMS

Pain

• TEARING, *drawing* pain. BURNING, rawness. In joints, bone.
• Soreness of parts lain on. As if broken, crushed. Sore all over.

Locations

• *Low back*: STIFF, crampy pain in kidney area, radiates to abdomen. < lying on the back > lying on painless side. Sacral pain.
• Sciatica < coughing, lying on back.
• *Neck*: Tension, torticollis drawn to the right < bending the head back > bending head forward.
• *Coccyx*: Drawing, bruised pain.
• *Hip*: Dislocation, inflammation, extends down or into abdomen.

Associated

• CONTRACTION and shortening of flexor tendons and muscles.
• STIFFNESS. N*eed to stretch*, bend, or crack joints.
• Feeling of shortening of muscles and ligaments.
• Joint deformity, tissue hardening, *ankylosis* or joint deposits.
• RESTLESSNESS < at night, in bed, in sleep, *not* > *by motion*.
• WEAKNESS of muscles. Atrophy. Progressive paralysis of a part.
• Numbness of a single part; trembling, twitching, cramps.
• Cracking of joints, especially knee < walking.
• Weak ankles, hip joints, hands, or thumbs, which feel sprained.

Modalities

< MOTION, overlifting, SITTING, rising up from sitting, standing, stooping, stepping, grabbing hold of anything.
< DRY, COLD, *wind*, open air. *Clear weather*, weather changes.

19

CAUSTICUM HAHNEMANNI

< LYING, Lying on back, lying on the affected area (hip & thigh pain), *lying on the painless side.*
< Getting wet or after bathing.
< *Evening,* 3-4 a.m. Right side. Night (hip pain). Menses.
> WARMTH, *warmth of the bed,* warm air. Gentle motion.
> DAMP, WET WEATHER.

▼ **SYMPTOM PROFILE**

Psychological
• Effects of CHRONIC SUFFERING. *Fears something will happen.* Guilt.
• Sympathetic and sensitive to injustice. Rebels against authority.
• Idealist, but becomes depressed, cynical, critical, contradictory.
• Forgetful; checking and re-checking.

Metabolic
• CHILLY. Effects of overwork, sleep loss, long caring for the sick.
• Progressive weakness. Sudden faintness. Emaciation.
• Warts on fingers. Sallow complexion. *Ill effects of burns or scars.*
• Antidotes mercury and lead. Antidoted by coffee, vinegar.

▼ **DOSAGE**

Potency
• 3rd to 30th in joint conditions.

Repetition
• Single dose, repeated when symptoms call for it.

▼ **CLINICAL CONDITIONS**

Musculoskeletal • Adhesions, scar tissue • Arthritic deformity
• Arthritis (chronic stages) • Carpal tunnel syndrome • Coccyx pain
• Dupuytren's contracture • Exostoses, osteophytes • Fibromyalgia
• Hip joint disease • Low back pain • Myalgia • Rheumatism
• Sciatica • Spasm • Tendonitis • TMJ disorders • Torticollis
• Writer's cramp.
Nervous System: • Bell's palsy / facial paralysis • Lead poisoning
• Meniere's disease • Multiple sclerosis • Neuralgia • Paralysis
• Parkinson's disease • Restless leg syndrome • Tremors.

CHAMOMILLA

German Chamomile

▼ KEYNOTES

➤ Joint inflammation or neuralgia with SPASM, NUMBNESS.
➤ Extreme pain with restlessness. Paralytic WEAKNESS with pain.
➤ < NIGHT, motion, heat of the bed. ANGER, irritability.

▼ JOINT AND NEURALGIC SYMPTOMS

Pain
• TEARING, drawing, stinging pains, seem unbearably intense.
• Pain, neuralgia, or any other complaint *coming on after* ANGER.

Locations
• NECK: Stiff, tense muscles with tearing pain.
• LOW BACK: Contractive or bruised pain radiating to abdomen, genital area < stooping, lying, menses. Feels bruised.
  < *Night, driving person out of bed*. Must walk about. Stiffness on sitting.
• Sacrum pain, radiating to the thighs or gut < menses, night.
• SCIATICA: Tearing pain from buttocks to feet with cramps, stiffness, weakness, heaviness < rising, stretching.
• *Lower limbs*: Hip pain < night or lying on opposite side. Stiffness in thighs. Pain in knee, calf > drawing the limbs up.
  CRAMPS in legs. Cracking of knee joint. Foot pain < motion. Paralytic weakness of feet at night. Ankles give way during the day. Soles burning; puts them out of bed at night. *Restless legs at night*.
• *Upper limbs*: Pain in shoulders, down arms. Arms numb, feel asleep < *trying to grasp anything*. Cold hands, sweaty palms. Swollen fingers.

Associated
• *Numbness*, SPASM, cramps. Stiffness, mainly from spasm.
• WEAKNESS, weariness as if paralyzed. Lame. No power in limbs.
• RESTLESSNESS; no position offers relief. Tosses about in bed.
• HOT SWEATS, which relieve < in sleep. Feels hot with pain. Thirst.
• Joints sore, feel bruised. Cracking joints. Jerking of limbs.
• STRETCHING, twisting, yawning. *Stretching out and drawing up limbs*.

Modalities
< MOTION, walking; yet pain forces him to move restlessly.

MATRICARIA CHAMOMILLA

< Stretching out the painful limb (though has the urge to).
< COLD, open air, *wind*, dry weather, cloudy weather.
< Heat, *getting warm in bed*. LYING on the painless side. Stretching.
< NIGHT. Touch. After anger. Pain < COFFEE.
> Warm, wet weather. Sweating. Change of position. Rising up.
> Cold compresses.

▼ SYMPTOM PROFILE

Psychological
- Extreme IRRITABILITY, tantrums, quarrelsome. Effects of anger.
- Hypersensitive, restless, complaining and whining, impatient.
- Aversion to *touch*, to interference, to being spoken to.
- Crying in sleep (adult or child). *Emotions felt in the stomach.*

Metabolic
- *Oversensitive to pain* or low pain threshold. Insomnia from pain.
- *Hot* and thirsty. One cheek red, the other pale.
- Spasms, cramps. Dysmenorrhea.

Pediatrics
- Primary remedy for teething, infantile colic, earache, diarrheas.
- ANGRY, whining, *demanding*. Capricious. Wants to be carried.

▼ DOSAGE

Potency
- 6, 12, or 30 in local conditions. Higher if emotions correspond.

Repetition
- Repeat until there is a response to the remedy (within three doses).

▼ CLINICAL CONDITIONS

- Arthritic or rheumatic *pain* < night • Brachial neuralgia • Cramps
- Facial neuralgia • Gout • Low back pain • Lumbar neuralgia
- Neuralgias • Numbness (paresthesias) of limbs • Paralysis
- Restless leg syndrome • Rheumatism • Sciatica • Spasms.

CHELIDONIUM

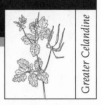

Greater Celandine

▼ KEYNOTES

➤ RIGHT thoracic or shoulder pain. HEAVY, stiff, lame, numb limbs.
➤ < MOTION, TOUCH, 4 p.m. and 4 a.m. > Heat, deep pressure.
➤ Associated LIVER disorders. Right-sided headache with vomiting.

▼ MUSCULOSKELETAL SYMPTOMS

Pain
• Sharp: STITCHING, tearing, shooting or PRESSING, "as if broken."
• Shooting backward from abdomen to back.

Location
• *Neck*: Pain, stiffness of RIGHT neck with head drawn to the side. Heaviness and tension in trapezius ①. Cold neck and occiput.
• RIGHT SHOULDER: Pain into arm with *stiffness in wrist* and arm. ②
• *Thorax*: Tearing pain in mid-thorax (T5-T8), extends through to breastbone. Thoracic neuralgia with stitches < inspiration.
• Pain at LOWER EDGE OF RIGHT SCAPULA ③, under scapula.
• *Low back*, RIGHT-sided sciatica; hip, knee, or heel rheumatism. ④

Headache
• Right occiput to frontal area and eye ⑤ with tearing, nausea, and bilious vomiting < warmth, motion > after vomiting.

Associated
• HEAVINESS of the part. As if paralyzed or lame. *Stiffness* of joints.
• Numbness of the limbs. Chills in the spine.
• Coldness of the tips of fingers. Icy coldness of the *right foot*.
• Secondary to, or associated with LIVER or *gall bladder* disorders. ⑥
• Perspiration without relief. Nausea and sweats with pain.

Modalities
< MOTION, change of position, deep breath. RIGHT SIDE.
< Bending back or forward, turning, stooping, rising up.
< WEATHER CHANGES, winds, 4 p.m., 4 a.m. (or earlier), sleep.

CHELIDONIUM MAJUS

< TOUCH or *pressure on the spine*. Lying on right side.
> Warmth, *hot applications* (except for headaches), deep pressure.
> Eating (headache and abdominal symptoms). Evening.

▼ **SYMPTOM PROFILE**

Psychological
- Domineering. Strong-minded, rational, skeptical.
- GUILT. Anxiety about health, death. Great irritability and anger.
- *Lethargic*: Mental depression, slow speech, thoughts, movement.
- Aversion to any mental or physical effort or activity.

Liver
- Inflammation or congestion of the liver. Right lobe of the liver.
- High cholesterol. JAUNDICE. Yellow tongue with imprints of teeth.

Digestive
- Gastralgia: Craves HOT DRINKS and milk, which relieve.
- Pain radiates to the right lower shoulder blade > EATING.
- Yellow or clay-colored stools; diarrhea and/or constipation.

Respiratory
- Right lung: coughs, asthma, pleurodynia, pneumonia.

▼ **DOSAGE**

Potency
- Lower potencies: 3rd to 12th.

Repetition
- Short-acting remedy.
- Can be repeated frequently.

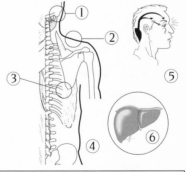

▼ **CLINICAL CONDITIONS**

- Brachial neuralgia • Bursitis • Facial neuralgia • Liver disorders
- Migraine headache (right side) • Rheumatism • Sciatica
- Shoulder pain • Tendonitis • Thoracic neuralgia • Torticollis.

CIMICIFUGA

Black Cohosh

▼ KEYNOTES

➤ Spine, NECK: Aching, shooting pains, *stiffness*, tension, *heaviness*.
➤ MUSCLE SPASMS, twitches < cold, damp > warmth, pressure.
➤ Anxiety and depression + uterine or ovarian problems.

▼ MUSCULOSKELETAL SYMPTOMS

Pain

• RADIATING, shooting, sharp. Violent ACHING. Like electric shocks.
• Cold, damp, or emotions bring on an attack of rheumatism.

Locations

• Affinity to large muscles; rheumatism, myalgia, fibromyalgia.
• *Head*: Headache from occiput to vertex, and above the right eye. ①
  < menses or instead of menses. Opening and shutting sensation.
• *Neck*: Drawing pain. STIFFNESS, contraction. Torticollis, head pulled
  back < draft ②. Pains into the left arm; feels bound to the side.③
• *Thoracic*: Upper three thoracic vertebrae ④ very sensitive to touch.
  Drawing mid-thoracic pain < bending forward or backward.
• *Lumbar*, sacral or sacro-iliac pain with radiation to FRONT OF
  THIGHS ⑤, through hips or around body. Pelvic pain, hip to hip.
  < Motion, touch, a.m. Violent aching. Weak & trembling type pain.
• *Feet*: Achilles tendonitis < walking, evening. Aching and stiff.

Associated

• SPASM of large muscles. *Cramps*. Twitching and jerking of limbs.
• STIFFNESS, contraction, *heaviness*. Feels *sore and bruised all over*.
• *Muscular soreness* < exertion. Muscular rheumatism and fatigue.
• *Spine sensitive* to the touch ⑥. Nausea from pressure in upper spine.
• RESTLESSNESS, trembling. Parts lain on go to sleep.
• Ovarian/uterine conditions alternate with joint/muscle pain. ⑦
• MENTAL SYMPTOMS alternate with rheumatic problems.

Modalities

< COLD, DAMP, *drafts*. Left side (except the head).
< MOTION, touch. During *menses*. Evening, *night*. MORNING.
< Menopause, puberty, pregnancy, childbirth. *Pressure* (tender spine)

CIMICIFUGA RACEMOSA

> Warmth, *wrapping up warmly* (except head), *open air*, eating.
> PRESSURE (back, head pain); in upper spine may cause nausea.
> Continued motion, REST,

▼ SYMPTOM PROFILE

Psychological

• DEPRESSION; as if a dark cloud encircles her, as if imprisoned.
• *Sighing*. Speaks in sighs. *Weeping*. Tears and laughter alternate.
• ANXIOUS, fidgety. Irrational fears. Fear of *insanity, death*, sleep.
• TALKATIVE, jumping from one subject to another. Excitable.
• Mental symptoms all < menses and > *during an attack of arthritis*.

Metabolic

• CHILLY but > open air. Craves cold drinks.
• Hypersensitive to noise, light. *Insomnia* from muscular pain.

Cardiovascular

• Rheumatism of chest ⑧. Angina-like symptoms on left side.

Female

• Spasmodic dysmenorrhea, PMS, menopause, pregnancy (fear, cramps). Uterine displacements, left ovarian problems.

▼ DOSAGE

Potency

• 3rd to 30th or higher.

Repetition

• Can be repeated frequently.

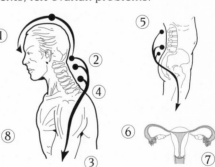

▼ CLINICAL CONDITIONS

• Achilles tendonitis (with stiffness, aching < walking)
• Brachial neuralgia • Fibromyalgia (Fibrositis) • Low back pain
• Lumbar neuralgia • Migraine • Myalgia • Myositis • Neuralgia
• Rheumatism • Sciatica • Tension headache.   .

COCCULUS

Indian Cockle

▼ KEYNOTES

➤ Headache with WEAK muscles, numbness, trembling. Vomiting.

➤ Rheumatism with cracking joints, stiffness < motion, yawning.

➤ < Noise, light, sleep loss, motion, talking, eating, jarring, menses.

▼ HEADACHE SYMPTOMS

Pain

• TEARING, throbbing. Constrictive or PRESSING. Pulsating pain.

• *Causes*: Loss of sleep. Mental strain. Emotional stress. After injury, from the sun. *Motion or travel.* Onset during menses, evenings.

Location

• OCCIPUT, radiating into the eyes. Forehead pain.

• Radiates to the neck, or *down the spine.*

Associated

• Many associated neurological symptoms. *Unique sensations include:*

— Hollowness or *emptiness* in the head, chest, or abdomen.

— Head as if separated from the body.

— Occiput *as if opening and shutting.* Shaking, rolling inside head.

• *Nausea & VOMITING, from *motion* or after food or drink < sight or smell of food. Associated vertigo or tinnitus.

• *Extreme* WEAKNESS; neck so weak, cannot hold head up; legs too weak to stand; too weak to speak.

• HEAVINESS of head > by bending backward.

• TREMBLING of hands on grasping or raising them. Cramps.

• Migrating NUMBNESS. Numbness of hands, *alternating sides* or hands alternating with the feet. Hands alternatively hot and cold.

• Nodding, shaking motions of head. ALL SENSES OVERSENSITIVE.

Modalities

< Noise (even causes vomiting), odors, cold, excitement.

< MOTION, motion of eyes, walking, riding (bumpy ride), JARRING.

< TALKING, touch. After sleep, open air, or cold wind.

< Eating and drinking, coffee or tea, tobacco. LOSS OF SLEEP.

23

COCCULUS INDICUS

< Lying on back of the head, during light. Menses.
> Warmth, quiet, *lying on the side*, or in bed.

▼ Joint Symptoms
- Painful CRACKING OF JOINTS. Painful STIFFNESS.
- *Rheumatism* from joint to joint with tenderness, swelling, stiffness.
- *Neck*: Pain and stiffness < moving the neck, yawning. Weakness of neck muscles with heaviness of the head.
- *Low back*: Paralytic pain, spasm < motion, cold, menses. Anxiety.
- *Shoulders* stiff, aching < rest, raising arm. Pains *like wires in arms*.
- *Knees*: CRACKING on motion. *Inflammation*, swelling, stitching pain.
- *Hands* fall asleep or are numb, alternating sides or with feet.
- *Feet*: Soles of feet asleep or numb. COLD FEET (with hot cheeks).

▼ Symptom Profile
Psychological
- CONFUSED and disoriented. Takes a long time answering questions or thinking. Dreamy, lost in their own sad thoughts.
- Worry, *anxiety about health of others*; sympathetic. GUILT, remorse.
- ANGER, easily offended, upset by rudeness of others.
- Talkative, joking and singing. Fear of death or impending disaster.

Female
- Dysmenorrhea, that is weakening. Menstrual headache.

▼ Dosage
Potency
- 30th to 200th.

Repetition
- Occasional single dose may be adequate.

▼ Clinical Conditions

• Brachial neuralgia • Headache • Knee rheumatism • Migraine • Motion sickness • Nausea of pregnancy • Parkinson's disease • Rheumatism • Shoulder bursitis • Vertigo.

COLCHICUM

Meadow Saffron

▼ KEYNOTES

➤ Acute arthritis or gout of small joints. WEAK, CHILLY, RESTLESS.
➤ Sore, stiff, swollen joints: Pale and puffy or red hot. *Wandering pain.*
➤ < MOTION, touch, night, COLD, damp, jarring > Sitting, stooping.

▼ MUSCULOSKELETAL SYMPTOMS

Pain
- *Bruised* SORENESS. Extreme tenderness.
- *Wandering* pains, from joint to joint. Go from *left to right.*
- Deep bone pain when the weather is cold.
- Electric vibration-like pains throughout the body.

Location
- Arthritis of small joints: fingers and toes, wrists, ankles, but also the shoulder and knee.
- Pain travels from below upward, above downward or across.
- *Upper limb*: Paralytic pain in arms, so painful that one cannot grasp an object firmly. Pains in arms extend into finger joints.
- *Lower limb*: Pain in legs, extending to toes. Leg cramps. SWOLLEN FEET. Foot cramps, pain in heels, soles, Achilles tendon.

Associated
- *Stiffness, weak and powerless*, as if paralyzed. EXTREME EXHAUSTION.
- Joints SWOLLEN, PUFFY, PALE or RED HOT. Swollen hands & feet.
- Large joints red, hot; small joints stiff and numb. CHILLY overall.
- Tingling, prickling, or numbness < fingertips.
- Rheumatism travels from the joints to the heart. High uric acid.
- NODOSITIES of the fingers. Bunions or gout of the big toe.
- Extreme RESTLESSNESS in all limbs.

Modalities
< Least MOTION (like Bryonia), walking, *exertion.* JARRING.
< Stretching out, straightening, or sitting erect.
< Hypersensitive to TOUCH, pressure, noise, *smells.*
< COLD, *damp, weather changes*, autumn, heat of the summer. *Night.*

24

COLCHICUM AUTUMNALE

< Getting wet or chilled. Getting the feet wet.
< From insomnia. From suppressed perspiration.
< Physical or mental overexertion, overstudy.
> SITTING, rest, standing. STOOPING or *sitting bent*. Bending double.
> Warmth or wrapping up, but overheating or hot air may WORSEN.

▼ SYMPTOM PROFILE

Psychological
- Extreme *irritability*. Dissatisfied.
- Oversensitive; disturbed by all sense impressions: light, sound.
- Very upset by BAD MANNERS OF OTHERS, by negative acts.
- Intellectual overwork, late nights. Sad. Weak memory.

Metabolic
- Fatigue. WEAKNESS of whole body; unable to move.
- Sedentary. Delicate and long-suffering individual.
- CHILLY, cold externally and internally. Sweats. Increased libido.

Digestive System
- Extreme distention, flatulence. Colic. Coldness in the abdomen.
- Diarrhea with jelly-like stools. *Mucus colitis*.
- NAUSEA from smells and odors.

Cardiovascular
- Valvular heart disease or pericarditis after rheumatism.
- Chest feels squeezed by a tight bandage. Pain in sternum.

▼ DOSAGE

Potency
- 3rd to 30th.

Repetition
- Requires frequent repetition when given in lower potencies.

▼ CLINICAL CONDITIONS

- Arthritis of small joints • Gout • Podagra • Rheumatism
- Rheumatoid arthritis (initial stages)
- Subacute or chronic swelling and inflammation.

COLOCYNTHIS

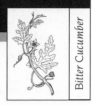

Bitter Cucumber

▼ **KEYNOTES**

➤ Acute or recent neuralgia, sciatica, or pain syndromes.

➤ *Vise-like* pain, with SPASM, cramps. Anger with the pain.

➤ < MOTION, touch, pressure, night > Doubling up, heat.

▼ **MUSCULOSKELETAL SYMPTOMS**

Pain

• NEURALGIC pain: sharp, *shooting*, lightning-like, tearing, or drawing.

• VISE or *band-like* pain. CRAMPING and griping. Deep bone pain.

• Recurrent episodes (every 15 minutes or more) of pain, SPASMS.

Location

• *Neck*: Intense muscle pain. Tenderness of vertebrae, with neuralgia on pressure of C1 to C3. STIFFNESS, drawing pain < turning.

• *Low back*: Severe stitches radiating into the thigh, buttock. Sacral pain shooting to the hip and down the back of the leg.

• *Sciatica*: Pain from posterior thigh and outside of left hip radiating to knees, ankle, or heel. Pain settles behind knee. Must limp. < 1st motion > continued motion < long continued motion. Heat first relieves, then later worsens.

• *Hip*: Inflammation, swelling in the buttock. Pain from hip to hip, radiates to knee and calf. Pain on motion or rotating leg inward. As if screwed in a vise. < motion, touch > rest, warmth of bed.

• *Arm*: Right shoulder, elbow or fingers sore and painful, stiff, swollen < motion, pressure. Restless limbs. Cramping in hands.

Associated

• Sudden or clutching SPASMS causing one to cry out or contort.

• Pain in limbs is followed by NUMBNESS or partial paralysis.

• Joints are swollen, stiff, painful. TENDER to pressure, touch.

• Muscle, joint, or tendon contracture or shortening with the pain.

• RESTLESS, but tries to control it. Restless at night.

• ANGER and irritability with the pain. Screams in pain. Nausea.

• WEAKNESS or faintness during or after the pain.

CITRULLUS COLOCYNTHIS

Modalities

< TOUCH (or pressure in chronic), cold, drafts, night, in bed.

< MOTION, lying, sitting, standing, walking, rotation (no position relieves). Lying on painless side.

< ANGER, emotional upset, excitement, left or *right side*. 4-5 p.m.

> BENDING DOUBLE. Flexing the leg on abdomen. *Lying on painful side* or on abdomen, lying with the head bent forward.

> HEAT (though heat may aggravate sciatica), WARMTH of bed, air.

> *Hard pressure*. REST (may sometimes be worse with rest).

▼ SYMPTOM PROFILE

Psychological

• IRRITABLE, impatient, easily offended < being questioned.

• *Effects of anger*, indignation, or humiliation resulting in spasms, cramps, or neuralgia.

• Taciturn, silent — disinclined to talk. Wants solitude.

Metabolic

• Obese, sedentary. Remedy antidoted by coffee. Antidotes lead.

Abdomen

• Abdominal pain or cramps < eating or drinking > doubling up, heat, pressure and > after stool.

• Diarrheas or colitis, kidney, ovarian, or gall bladder colic.

▼ DOSAGE

· Potency

• 3rd to 200th potency.

Repetition

• Single doses as required. A dose after the attack has subsided.

▼ CLINICAL CONDITIONS

> • Brachial neuralgia • Coccyx pain • Headache • Hip dislocation
> • Hip joint disease • Low back pain • Neck problems / Torticollis
> • Nerve root lesions • Neuralgia • Sacroiliac pain • Sciatica
> • Spasms, cramps • Thoracic neuralgia • Trigeminal neuralgia.

DULCAMARA

Bittersweet

▼ KEYNOTES

➤ Acute or subacute rheumatism brought on by DAMP conditions.
➤ Stiff, cold, painful joints alternate with skin eruptions or diarrhea.
➤ < COLD, DAMP, rest, night > Warmth, dry, continued MOTION.

▼ MUSCULOSKELETAL SYMPTOMS

Pain
• Drawing, tearing, stitching, or prickling pains. Shooting pain.

Location
• Rheumatism, especially of *muscles*; muscular soreness.
• *Low back* pain, lameness, *as if stooping too long*. Stitches and tension on motion < stooping, rest, cold, deep breath > pressure. Shooting pains, radiate to thighs. CHILLS IN SPINE.
• *Sciatica* < sitting, COLD > motion, walking.
• *Neck*: STIFFNESS < cold, damp, turning. Dull pain into shoulders.
• *Arms*: Paralysis of arms with COLDNESS < rest > motion. Swelling of hands, wrist. Stiffness of fingers on outstretching arm.
• *Legs*: Stitching pain in thighs or in legs < rest, sitting > walking. Cramps in ankles. Burning feet.

Causes
• Ailments due to DAMP and COLD living or working conditions.
• Getting the feet wet or cold; chilling of the face (neuralgia).
• Rheumatism from suppression of perspiration or *skin eruptions*.
• Chilling after being overheated or after sweating.

Associated
• Joints inflamed, red, swollen, tender, with dry hot skin.
• STIFFNESS, swelling, twitching.
• Rheumatism alternating with diarrhea or skin disease.
• COLDNESS *of painful areas*. Burning feet < night, lying, cold.

Modalities
< COLD or DAMP: environments, houses, cellars, air conditioning.
< Wet or rainy weather. Getting wet or chilled. Cold air, drafts.

DULCAMARA

< *Change from warm to cold or dry to damp.* Autumn. NIGHT.
< When at REST, sitting.
> *Warm, dry* weather or environment. Radiant heat, warm bed.
> MOTION, movement of the area, continued motion, walking.
> Pressure, warm applications.

▼ SYMPTOM PROFILE

Psychological
• Domineering, controlling, possessive, quarrelsome. Abusive.
• *Demands and then rejects things.* Depressed, confused, poor memory.
• Anxiety about the future, about others.

Metabolic
• CHILLY < cold or damp. *Feet freezing cold.* Swollen glands. Edema.

Respiratory
• Frequent colds, chronic sinus, ear catarrh, hay fever, allergies, or asthma: caused by *damp and cold*, with profuse discharges.

Digestive
• Diarrhea in cold, damp. Simultaneous vomiting.

Urinary
• Cystitis or incontinence from damp, cold.

Skin
• Eruptions alternate with rheumatism or diarrhea.
• Eczema or impetigo, oral or genital herpes, hives, URTICARIA.
• Large *fleshy warts* on hands and fingers.

▼ DOSAGE

Potency
• 3rd to 30th.

Repetition
• May be repeated in lower potencies.

▼ CLINICAL CONDITIONS

> • Arthritis • Cervical rheumatism • Exostosis (tibia, forearm) • Gout
> • Headache • Low back pain • Myalgia • Myelitis • Neuritis, neuralgia
> • Paralysis • Rheumatism • Sciatica • Torticollis.

Note: *All conditions* caused by or much worse from COLD and DAMP.

FORMICA RUFA

Red Ants

▼ KEYNOTES

➤ Inflammation of joints and muscle. Nodosities, osteophytes.
➤ Sudden, erratic, shifting pains with excitability, RESTLESSNESS.
➤ < Motion, cold, damp > Warmth, rubbing, pressure. Easy fatigue.

▼ MUSCULOSKELETAL SYMPTOMS

Pain

• SUDDEN rheumatic pains, erratic and CHANGEABLE (24-48 hours).
• May shift from right to left or left to right.
• From overlifting, injury, cold weather, *suppression of foot sweat.*
• Muscles feel strained, as if torn at their sites of attachment.

Locations

• *Neck pain,* arm neuralgia < bending back, motion, sitting up > *heat.*
• Pain in the neck when chewing < on closing the jaws.
• Left elbow and wrist pain, or pain wanders from left or right.
• Left sacro-iliac pain. Low back pain.
• Rheumatic pain in knee joints < walking.

Associated

• RESTLESSNESS though < motion. Desires activity but too tired.
• EASY FATIGUE. Lethargy and need to lie down.
• Stiffness, CONTRACTION of joints.
• Hard *nodosities* around joints. *Osteophytosis,* exostoses.
• SKIN RASH. Red and itching. Vasculitis, hives (like ant bites).
• *Mental agitation,* excitability, buoyancy.
• In acute conditions, *profuse sweats which give no relief.*
• Numbness or falling asleep of hands or feet. Cramps of feet.
• Weakness of lower limbs.
• *Gout* or high uric acid.

Modalities

< MOTION. COLD, cold water, damp, *before snowfall.* Sitting. *Right side.*
> PRESSURE. HEAT. Massage. Rest, lying. After midnight.

FORMICA RUFA

▼ SYMPTOM PROFILE

Psychological
- Mentally ACTIVE, cheerful. Restless, EXCITABLE, nervous.
- Desires activity but *too exhausted*. Weakened memory < evening.
- Depression with apathy, dejection, irritability.
- < Effects of bad news, humiliation. *Dwells on past sad events*.
- Dreams of funerals, coffins or sexual dreams.

ENT
- NASAL POLYPS. Nasal obstruction. Weak vision. *Rheumatic iritis*.

Nervous System
- Headache all day, afternoon > pressure. Stroke. Paralysis.

Digestive
- Fetid, putrid diarrhea < waking or after breakfast. Umbilical pain.

Skin
- *Red, itching, burning*. Flat HIVES < cold water. Wounds that atrophy.

Urinary
- Albuminuria. Frequent urination; phosphates, urates. Fetid odor.

▼ DOSAGE

Potency
- Low potency: 3, 6, 12, 30, or 200.

Repetition
- Can be repeated in lower potencies as symptoms require.

▼ CLINICAL CONDITIONS

Joints
- Facial neuralgia after extraction or decay • Gout
- Lupus and connective tissue disorders • Migratory arthritis
- Old injuries, strains, or dislocations • Osteoarthritis
- Osteophytes • Reiter's syndrome • Rheumatism
- Sacroiliac arthritis • TMJ problems.

Bone
- Bone tumors (jaw, lower extremities) • Exostosis • Osteitis
- Osteosarcoma • Periostitis (acute and chronic) • Rickets.

GELSEMIUM

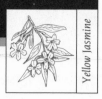

Yellow Jasmine

▼ KEYNOTES

❋➤   Dull, listless, apathetic. Vertigo, weakness, trembling.
➤ Dull headache with blurred vision at onset.
➤ < Warm wet weather, mental or physical exertion, heat, sun.

▼ HEADACHE SYMPTOMS

Pain

• DULL, aching, heaviness. B*and-like constriction*.
• BURSTING pain in eyes and forehead.
• Insidious onset. B*lurring of vision*, double vision. Noise sensitivity.

Location

• Headache originating in the CERVICAL SPINE.
• *Occiput* extending to eyes, forehead, face, neck, clavicles, shoulder.

Associated

• *Causes*: Emotional upset, fright, grief, anger. Sun, storms, warm or cold damp weather, weather changes.
• Light-headed, faint, *dizziness*. HEAVY LIDS. *Heavy head*, heavy limbs.
• M*uscular weakness*, incoordination and awkwardness. *Trembling*.
• *Intoxicated feeling*. Drowsiness, lethargy, fatigue. Chills in the spine.
• Face dark red, flushed. Headache during colds or flu.
• *Cold feet, hot face*. Numbness.
• Neck and shoulders sore. Soreness of scalp.

Modalities

< *Cold* and DAMP, or WARM WET WEATHER, before storms, fog.
< *Heat*, heat of the *sun*. Summer.
< Bad news, frights or fear, anticipation, worry, mental exertion.
< *Motion or exertion*.
< LYING or letting the head hang low.
< Light, noise, 10 a.m., tobacco smoke.
> Profuse urination or perspiration, *pressure*.
> *Lying with head raised on a pillow*. Rest, lying down, sleep.
> Alcohol, vomiting. Closing the eyes.

GELSEMIUM SEMPERVIRENS

▼ MUSCULOSKELETAL SYMPTOMS

- *Neck*: Bruised pain in the neck, under the left shoulder blade, and in the sternomastoid muscle. Sense of contraction of the right side. Stiffness, lameness. Tender, sensitive to pressure.
- *Sciatica*: Burning pain < rest, first motion, night. Pain in the sole of the foot on walking. Legs feel powerless, weak.
- *Limbs* feel weak, tired, HEAVY. Numbness. Paralysis, gradual loss of muscular control. Coldness of the hands and feet.
- *Low back*: Dull aching in lumbar and sacral spine. Unable to walk.

▼ SYMPTOM PROFILE

Psychological
- Confused, DULL, apathetic. Loss of will. *Wants solitude and silence.*
- Unable to think. Weak and weary, lethargic.
- Stage fright. ANTICIPATION ANXIETY, apprehension and timidity.
- Excitable. Insomnia and sleep disorders.

▼ DOSAGE

Potency
- 6, 12, or 30.

Repetition
- Not a deep or long-acting remedy.
- Repeat frequently in acute conditions.

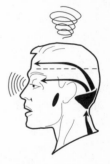

▼ CLINICAL CONDITIONS

Headache: • During colds or flu • Migraine headache • Sun headache • Tension or muscle contraction headache.
Nervous System: • Motor paralysis: of the eyes, throat, limbs • Multiple sclerosis • Myasthenia gravis • Parkinson's disease • Twitches, neuralgias, spasms.
Musculoskeletal: • Dupuytren's contracture • Myalgia • Neuralgia • Rheumatism • Spasms • Tic doloreux • Writer's cramp.

GNAPHALIUM

Sweet Everlasting

▼ KEYNOTES

➤ Specific for SCIATICA or neuralgia of the leg.
➤ Sharp pain, shooting down leg, alternating with NUMBNESS.
➤ < Motion, cold, damp > Drawing the limbs up.

▼ SCIATICA SYMPTOMS

Pain

• INTENSE, darting, or cutting sensations. Shooting pain.

Location

• Pain along entire length of the sciatic nerve and its large branches: into the hip, thigh, back of the thigh, foot, or toes. < Right side.
• Neuralgia of the front of the leg (crural neuralgia).

Associated

• NUMBNESS follows the pain or alternates with the pain.
• Sciatica with FORMICATION (crawling sensation).
• *Low back pain*: Chronic aching with NUMBNESS in the lumbar and lumbosacral area > lying on the back. Numbness of the thighs.
• Sensation of weight, heaviness in the pelvis.
• CRAMP in the calves, feet, or ankles < at night in bed.
• Chronic muscular rheumatism of the back and neck.
• Rheumatism of the ankles or toes. Gout of the toes.
• Exercise is very fatiguing from numbness in the legs.
• Diarrhea with joint problems.
• Joints feel *as if they are lacking oil*, i.e., dry and creaky.

Modalities

< MOTION. Stepping, walking. Stretching.
< Lying down.
< *Cold and damp*. Wet weather. Night. *Right side*.
> Drawing limbs up (flexing the leg onto the abdomen).
> Sitting in a chair.

29

GNAPHALIUM POLYCEPHALUM

▼ **SYMPTOM PROFILE**

Psychological
- Irritable and morose.
- Nervous and restless at night.
- Weakness, worse in the morning on waking.
- Sleep is unrefreshed.

Head
- Vertigo after rising.
- Dull pain in the back of the head, sense of fullness > cold bathing.

Digestive
- NAUSEA and vomiting. Nausea of pregnancy. *Nausea during diarrhea.*
- Diarrhea and cramps. Watery, offensive, light-colored.

Female
- Dysmenorrhea. Breast tumors or nodules. Stitching pains.

Male
- Increased sexual desire. Erection on waking. Prostatic irritation.

▼ **DOSAGE**

Potency
- 3rd to 30th potency.

Repetition
- Repeat as needed according to symptoms.

▼ **CLINICAL CONDITIONS**

- Anterior leg neuralgia • Brachial neuralgia • Eye pain
- Facial neuralgia • Gout (feet) • Headache • Leg cramps
- Low back pain • Rheumatism of knees, legs, ankles, toes • Sciatica.

GUAIACUM

Lignum Vitae

▼ KEYNOTES

➤ Arthritis and joint inflammation with tearing, stitching, burning.
➤ Stiffness, contraction of tendons, deformity of joints.
➤ < MOTION and HEAT, cold and damp > Cold applications.

▼ MUSCULOSKELETAL SYMPTOMS

Pain

• Tearing, STITCHING, pressing, or *contractive* pain.
• Burning pain and heat. Growing pains.

Location

• *Spine*: One-sided stiffness of the whole back, from neck to sacrum.
• *Neck*: Aching or stitching. STIFFNESS < left side, motion, cold.
• *Thorax*: Contractive pain between the scapulae < deep breathing.
• *Low back* pain with stiffness.
• *Upper extremity*: Stiff and sore shoulders, arms. W*rist affinity*, carpal tunnel syndrome. Pain elbow to wrist. Fingers curved and stiff.
• *Lower extremity*: Knee and ankle arthritis.

Associated

• CONTRACTION, tightness, tension. *Shortening* of muscles, of flexor tendons, *hamstrings*. Joint deformity. Exostoses.
• STIFFNESS: *Feels need to stretch or yawn*, which relieves.
• BURNING and heat in affected area or whole limb.
• Weakness, weariness in arms, thighs. Muscular atrophy.
• Prickling in the buttocks as if sitting on needles.
• Pain, itching, crawling in the thighs while seated.
• Swollen joints. Sensitive to touch.

Modalities

< MOTION, exertion, sitting. Pressure (may relieve), open air.
< HEAT, heat of the bed, *left side*. *Touch*. Cold or damp, wet weather.
< Evening and morning. From 6 p.m. to 4 a.m.— especially the neck.
> COLD APPLICATIONS. *Stretching*, yawning. Rubbing. Indoors.

30 •

GUAIACUM OFFICINALE

▼ **SYMPTOM PROFILE**

Psychological
- Critical, HATEFUL, quarrelsome. Rigid and inflexible. Stubborn.
- Dull, sluggish. WEAK MEMORY, especially for names.

Metabolic
- CHILLY, yet joint problems > from cold and < heat.
- Profuse perspiration. Night sweats.
- OFFENSIVENESS of sweat and all other secretions.
- Craves apples, which > stomach problems.
- Headache and chest pain < sitting, standing > pressure, walking.

Sleep
- Insomnia, restless sleep. Frequent waking with sensation of falling or nightmares. Cries out in sleep. Dreams of struggle, falls.

Throat
- Tonsillitis, sore throat: stiff, dry, BURNING, stitching.

▼ **DOSAGE**

Potency
- Low potencies: 3, 6, 12, or 30.

Repetition
- A deep-acting remedy, but can be repeated often.

▼ **CLINICAL CONDITIONS**

Musculoskeletal
- Arthritis • Arthritis deformans • Arthritis or rheumatism after tonsillitis or other infections • Bone disease • Carpal tunnel syndrome • Dupuytren's contracture • Frozen shoulder • Gout • Growing pains (in children who grow too rapidly) • Joint deformity • Low back pain • Osteoarthritis • Osteomalacia • Osteophytosis • Rheumatism • Tendonitis • Torticollis.

Nervous System
- Brachial neuralgia • Headache • Neuralgia • Sciatica (> warmth).

HECLA LAVA

Volcanic Ash

▼ KEYNOTES

➤ Osteophytes, exostoses of small joints.
➤ Bone growths, tumors, cysts, exostoses of the long bones, head.
➤ Bone inflammation (osteitis), weakness, or metabolic disease.

▼ MUSCULOSKELETAL SYMPTOMS

Joint Conditions
• ARTHRITIC NODOSITIES.
• Myalgia of intercostal muscles.
• Hip joint disease.
• Hallux vulgus.
• Deformity or nodules of the fingers, toes.

Bone Conditions
• BONE TUMORS or exostoses, especially of the head, jaws, leg.
• Tumors of the TIBIA with severe continuous pain.
• Swollen and bulging thighs and legs. Exostoses of fingers.
• Bone inflammation: Osteitis, periostitis.
• Osteomalacia (Rickets). Osteitis deformans.
• Benign bone tumors.
• Osteosarcoma. Necrosis and destruction of bone.

Associated
• Painful bone tumors or nodosities *after injury.*
• Sleepiness and yawning.

Modalities
< Touch, pressure. Beginning of motion, sitting, rest. Left side.

Note: *Though not a frequently used remedy, Hecla should be considered as a powerful tool for reducing osteophytes, bone spurs (including calcaneal spurs), and exostoses, along with better known remedies like Calc fluor.*

31

HECLA LAVA

▼ **SYMPTOM PROFILE**

Face & Head

• FACE: *Neuralgia* from tooth decay, dental work or extraction. Extreme tenderness. Facial swelling. Cannot eat or sleep.
• HEAD: Headache from dental or bone disease. Tumors of the skull.
• TUMORS of the face, nose or *jaw* (upper or lower maxillary bones).
• EAR: Caries of mastoid bone. Exostosis in external meatus of ear.
• NOSE: Nasal polyps or tumors. Ulceration.
• *Swollen cervical glands*, like a string of pearls.
• Vertigo: everything goes up, down, and sideways.

Dental

• Dental ABSCESS with swelling, pus < pressure on teeth. Gumboil.
• Delayed or difficult dentition in malnourished children.
• Decay of teeth. TOOTHACHE. Pain or neuralgia *after extraction*.
• Chronic dental or jaw abscess. Chronic gingivitis. Fistula.

Other Areas

• Breast tumors or nodules. Diminished milk while nursing.
• Varicose veins. Nephritis. Inflammation of the kidneys or ureters.
• Black warts. Actinomycosis.

▼ **DOSAGE**

Potency

• Mainly used in low potency (3x - 6x) but 30c and 200c are effective.

Repetition

• Low potencies daily for several months in bone or joint pathology.

▼ **CLINICAL CONDITIONS**

• Arthritis deformans • Arthritic nodosities • Bone tumors or cysts
• Hip joint arthritis • Facial neuralgia • Exostoses • Intercostal myalgia • Osteitis • Osteitis deformans • Osteomalacia • Osteosarcoma
• Paget's disease • Periostitis • Rickets • Syphilis of the bones
• Tooth decay.

HYPERICUM

St. John's Wort

▼ KEYNOTES

➤ Injury to NERVES and nerve-rich tissue. Pains shoot UPWARD.
➤ Trauma of the SPINE, HEAD, COCCYX, fingertips. Tenderness.
➤ Neuralgia, sciatica, depression, or headache after injury. Shock.

▼ MUSCULOSKELETAL SYMPTOMS

Pain
- Sharp pains, SHOOT UPWARD from the site of injury.
- Intense, violent pains, appear and disappear gradually.

Location
- Pains shoot up the spine or limbs from the site of injury.
- Pain along the length of the nerve.
- Neck and spine SENSITIVE. Neck pain < slightest motion.

Associated
- Part EXCESSIVELY TENDER, painful and sore.
- Weakness and trembling. Jerking and twitching of muscles.
- Crawling, numbness, or burning.
- Mental shock or depression. Despair or sadness with the pain.

Modalities
< TOUCH, *motion*, exertion, jarring. Rising from sitting.
< Lying on the back. Sciatica < sitting.
< COLD, *cold weather* or air, damp. *Change of weather, fog*, storms.
> Bending backward, rubbing, rest.

▼ EXTERNAL USE

- Bleeding wounds, deep lacerations, puncture wounds.
- Burns, including sunburn.
- Dirty wounds or cuts, to prevent or heal infection.

▼ SYMPTOM PROFILE

Psychological
- *Depression* or mental weakness after injury, wounds, or surgery.
- After injury, sensation of the head being elongated or of being lifted high in the air with fear of falling from this height.

HYPERICUM PERFORATUM

▼ Clinical Conditions

Nervous System

- *Nerve trauma*: Injury to nerves, or to the *spine, head, coccyx.*
- Neuralgia: After wounds, surgery, amputation < weather changes.
- *Neuritis*: Head, chest, thoracic spine, if due to injury.
- *Sciatica* (from injury): Foot pain, weakness and trembling < sitting.
- Median or ulnar nerve injury or neuralgias.
- *Head*: Headache after head injury or falls on the buttocks, heels, or spine. Bursting pain on the vertex.
- *Concussion* • *Convulsions* after injury • *Vertigo*, dizziness after injury.

Trauma & Injury

- *Spinal sprains* or fracture • Lumbar puncture • SHOCK.
- *Coccyx pain*: From falls or blows, childbirth.
- Crushing injuries to the *fingers or toes.*
- Effects of PAST INJURIES to the above areas (use higher potency).
- Potential or actual *infection* from wounds, with pus formation.
- *Hemorrhage* from injuries, deep cuts, or lacerations.
- *Puncture wounds*, insect or animal bites (especially of the palms or soles), injections • Preventive for lockjaw / tetanus.
- *Dental work, surgery, or fracture* which damages or injures nerves.
- *Burns*: Including sunburn or radiation burns (external & internal).
- *Cicatrices*: For painful old scars (acts on the nerves, not on the scar).
- In severe wounds, preserves vitality of partially severed tissue.
- For antidoting the effects of radiation and EMF (electrical fields).
- Trauma to the eye, with severe pains.

▼ Dosage

Potency

- 6, 12, or 30. High potency for the effects of past injuries.
- External application: Use the same as you would with Calendula, or combine the two for a healing lotion.

Repetition

- Repeat frequently in acute or initial stages.
- Past nerve, spine, or head injuries: use high potency weekly.

IRS VERS

Blue Flag

▼ KEYNOTES

➤ Weekend headache / migraine preceded by visual disturbances.
➤ Acrid VOMITING. Pain < rest, evening, cold air > gentle motion.
➤ Onset from fatigue, resting after stress, sweets, stomach upset.

▼ HEADACHE SYMPTOMS

Onset

• Headache starts when relaxing, particularly after prolonged stress.
• *Weekly headache.* Onset every morning after breakfast or 2-3 a.m.
• VISUAL DISTURBANCES, blurring or blindness at the start. ①
• Heavy, sleepy, tired before headache commences.
• May vomit before pain actually begins.
• Causes: *Mental exhaustion.* Cold air. *After sweets.* Stomach upset.

Pain

• CONSTRICTIVE ②, band-like pain. *Pulsating, shooting,* fullness, heat.

Location

• FOREHEAD ③, TEMPLE ④ . *Right-sided* or alternating sides, but spreads to the whole head. Stitching in the occiput. ⑤
• Right temple to left occiput. Pain above the eye. ⑥

Associated

• Nausea and bitter, sour, or acrid VOMITING ⑦. Sour belching.
• BURNING pain in the pit of the stomach (pancreas area).
• Acidic and BURNING DIARRHEA.
• *Increased salivation.* Thick ropy saliva, drips from the mouth. ⑧
• Buzzing and roaring in the ears. Tinnitus. Vertigo.
• Much urination after attack of headache.

Modalities

< EVENING or night. 2-3 a.m. Weekly or periodically. SUNDAYS.
< *Lying or* RESTING, sitting, studying. First motion. *Violent motion or exertion.* Coughing, laughing. Cold air. Hot weather.
< RIGHT SIDE or *right to left.* Spring and fall. After breakfast.
> CONTINUED, GENTLE MOTION. Open air. Cold applications.

IRIS VERSICOLOR

Other Areas
- LOW BACK PAIN on motion or rising up. Cramping pain on right.
- SHOULDER tension and pain < motion or raising the arms.
- SCIATICA with pain in the *left* hip, to the knee and foot < motion.

▼ **SYMPTOM PROFILE**

Psychological
- *Depression and gloom.* Anxiety regarding the approaching illness.
- DULL and sluggish with the headache. Dreams of death, graves.
- Delicate, refined, nervous. Well-mannered. Sleepless with pain.

Metabolic
- Mental or sedentary workers. WEAKNESS, enervation, trembling.
- Affects the glands: Thyroid, pancreas, salivary glands, liver.

Throat
- BURNING, hot throat. Profuse flow of saliva. *Sweet taste.* Goiter.

Digestive
- SOUR or acrid VOMITING. Nausea. Heartburn. Hyperacidity.
- BURNING anywhere along the digestive tract; not > cold drinks.
- Burning eructations, sour and acrid belching.
- Watery, *burning* diarrhea. Enteritis. Rumbling and cramps.
- Inflammation of the pancreas. Diabetes.

Skin
- Psoriasis, shingles, eczema, impetigo, boils. Facial acne. Oily nose.

▼ **DOSAGE**

Potency
- 3x, 6x, up to the 30th.

Repetition
- Frequent repetitions during acute symptoms.

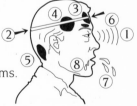

▼ **CLINICAL CONDITIONS**

- Facial neuralgia • Headache • Herpes zoster • Hip pain • Low back pain • Migraine • Neuralgia • Sciatica (left) • Shoulder rheumatism.

KALI CARB

K_2CO_3

Potassium Carbonate

▼ **KEYNOTES**

➤ STITCHING pains radiating up and down, into thighs, buttocks.
➤ Weakness & giving out of the back. Pain impedes breathing.
➤ < Standing, sitting erect, *bending back* > Stooping, lying, pressure.

▼ **LOW BACK SYMPTOMS**

Pain
• STITCHING, *sharp*, cutting. HEAVY, like a weight. Aching, drawing.
• As if it would break, as if torn. PRESSING inward. Burning.

Location
• Pains radiate *up and down the spine* from the low back.
• Extends downwards, radiates to the thighs, BUTTOCKS.

Associated
• WEAK BACK, muscles and lax ligaments. "GIVING OUT" feeling.
• Must lie down or lean on something. Must *walk stooped*.
• Pain impedes respiration. Cannot take a proper breath.
• Pulsation alternating with the pain.
• Twitching on stooping. Tickling sensations.
• Back and feet very sensitive to *touch*. Wants the back PRESSED.
• Pain *drives him out of bed in the morning*, at midnight, or at 3 a.m.
• Pains across the sacrum with stiffness of the back.

Causes
• Back pain after childbirth, miscarriage, during pregnancy, delivery.
• From INJURY or exertion. Everything seems to trigger a backache.

Modalities
< Standing, walking, sitting, exertion. BEING ERECT. During REST.
< *Bending backward*. Sudden motion (causes stitching pains).
< Breathing. TOUCH. *Lying on the painful side*. Right side.
< 3 a.m., morning on rising from bed. During or before MENSES.
< COLD, *drafts, damp*. Chilling after overheating. Weather changes.
> PRESSURE, rubbing. LYING ON THE BACK, on a hard surface.

34 •

KALI CARBONICUM

> MOTION (limbering up or easy motion). *Warmth*, dryness. Open air.
> STOOPING (standing, walking, or sitting bent forward).

▼ SYMPTOM PROFILE

Psychological
- Conservative, responsible, dutiful, moralistic, *possessive*, depressed.
- Fear of losing control. *Hypochondriacal* < when alone.
- Hypersensitive to pain, noise, touch.

Metabolic
- CHILLY < *cold in all forms*: cold wind, drinks, food, weather, drafts.
- Fat; flabby muscles; lax ligaments; tissues soft and puffy.
- Edema, fluid retention. Puffiness above eyes.
- WEAKNESS. *Perspires easily*. Sweating of feet. *Craves sweets*.
- Flushes of heat.

Digestive
- *Emotions felt in the stomach*. Excess flatulence. Constipation.

Chest
- Coughs, asthma, dyspnea. Pleurisy. Heart weakness and angina.

Female
- AMENORRHEA, infertility. Dysmenorrhea. Miscarriage. Problems after childbirth. Back pain associated with these conditions.

▼ DOSAGE

Potency
- Generally the 30c for musculoskeletal conditions.

Repetition
- Infrequent repetition. Single doses are often sufficient.
- High potencies not to be used in advanced rheumatism or gout.

▼ CLINICAL CONDITIONS

> - Backache after abortion, labor • Hip joint disease (right side)
> - Knee conditions • Low back pain • Migraine • Overstrain.

KALMIA

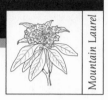

Mountain Laurel

▼ KEYNOTES

➤ RHEUMATISM or NEURALGIA, changes place rapidly.
➤ Numbness, weakness, trembling. Related heart or eye symptoms.
➤ Shooting pains that travel DOWNWARD < motion, cold, night.

▼ JOINT AND NERVE SYMPTOMS

Pain

• Sharp, sticking. SHOOT DOWNWARD, from the center outward, upper to lower. *Come and go gradually.* Changes place after rubbing.
• Aching, bruised. SORE, tender. BURNING and heat in the spine.

Location

• RAPIDLY CHANGING locations; from joint to joint; from upper limbs to lower limbs, with several joints affected.
• ALTERNATING AREAS: shoulder and hip, elbow and shoulder, etc.
• *Neck*: Pain radiating to shoulders, arms, fingers, face, head, or back.
• *Thorax*: Pain in upper thoracic or between shoulder blades, radiating into the shoulder, arm, or head. Cracking of vertebrae.
• *Low Back*: Aching and burning pain. Lameness < at night in bed.
• *Limbs*: Inflammation of literally any joint: wrist, fingers, hip, knee.
• Cracking and cramps of the elbow joint.
• *Headache*: Pain in the forehead extending to the eye and upper teeth < on waking, sunrise to sunset, in the sun, heat > cloudy weather.

Associated

• NUMBNESS, tingling, crawling before or after the pain.
• Joints are HOT, RED, and SWOLLEN. Stiffness. Cracking joints.
• Rheumatism with generalized, intense WEAKNESS.
• Neuralgia with local weakness, TREMBLING, or paralysis.
• Alternating or associated heart symptoms.
• Rheumatism alternates with skin eruptions.

Modalities

< Least MOTION, turning, bending forward or backward, exertion.
< Lying in bed. Looking down or *lying on the left*. LEFT SIDE. *Touch*.

KALMIA LATIFOLIA

< COLD or *getting chilled*. Wind. Weather changes. Open air. Damp.
< Evening or first part of the NIGHT. Winter. MENSES.
> Warmth, warm applications. Rest. *Lying on the back.*

▼ SYMPTOM PROFILE

Psychological
• Anxiety in the heart area with palpitations, chest pain, or dyspnea.
• IRRITABLE, angry, morose, silent. < Talking about others.
• Confusion, difficult concentration. Nightmares. Sleep-walking.

Eyes
• Rheumatic iritis, scleritis. *Stiffness of the eye.* Eye pain with the sun.
• Facial neuralgia with radiation into the right eye.

Cardiovascular
• Rheumatism affecting or alternating with HEART CONDITIONS.
• Bad effects of *tobacco*. Angina with PALPITATIONS. Hypertrophy.
• *Very slow pulse* (or may be rapid). Angina. Palpitations. Suffocation.

Kidney
• Nephritis. Loss of protein. Bright's disease.

▼ DOSAGE

Potency
• Low potency: 6 or 12.

Repetition
• Short-acting. Bears repetition well.

▼ CLINICAL CONDITIONS

Musculoskeletal
• Arthritis • Bone pains (night) • Carpal tunnel syndrome • Gout
• Headache • Low back pain • Lumbar neuralgia • Reiter's syndrome
• RHEUMATISM • Rheumatoid arthritis (arthritis, iritis, urethritis)
• Shoulder rheumatism • Tennis elbow • Thoracic pain.

Neurological
• Brachial neuralgia • Crural neuralgia • Headache from the sun
• Herpes zoster or neuralgia after suppression of eruption
• Intercostal neuralgia • NEURITIS • Sciatica • Ulnar neuritis.

LACHESIS

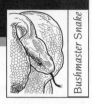

Bushmaster Snake

▼ KEYNOTES

➤ Migraine: forehead, temples, vertex. HEAT, flushes. Menopause.
➤ 1. Pressing   2. Cutting and stabbing   3. Pulsating or bursting.
➤ < MORNING, motion, sleep > Flow of discharges, lying, pressure.

▼ HEADACHE SYMPTOMS

Pain
- CUTTING, darting, STABBING, like a knife.
- PRESSING. Pressing *outward* < motion, walking, sitting > lying.
- PULSATING in sides, temple, on waking. Bursting. *Blood congestion.*
- *Burning pain.* Aching deep in the brain. Sudden, intense episodes.
- *Onset:* After sleep, mornings, with visual disturbances, dim vision,

Location
- FOREHEAD, or *above the eye,* extends to root of the NOSE, to the eyes, or backward to the occiput, even down the back.
- ONE-SIDED headache. *Left* or right-sided, or from right to left.
- TEMPLES or sides. Radiates to the shoulder, ear.
  Pain as if a piece cut out the parietal bone (side of the head).
- VERTEX: Burning, *heat.* Pain extends to jaw, side of the head, face.
- *Occiput:* extends to the eyes, forehead < closing the eyes.

Causes
- Emotional excitment. COLDS. Alcohol. Cold air. Smell of coffee
- During MENOPAUSE. Ovarian or uterine disease. From the SUN.

Associated
- Rushes of blood with HEAT in the head. Heaviness in the occiput.
- *Pale face.* Stiffness in the neck, or general stiffness.
- Regular attacks, every 8 to 10 days. Burning on vertex (menopause).
- VERTIGO: during the day < closing the eyes, walking > lying.
- Shocks, jerking of the head. Unable to raise the head in the a.m.
- Scalp very sensitive, sore. Occiput sore to touch < *pressure of pillow.*
- Heart difficulties with the headache. Palpitations.
- COLD, chilliness in the head (especially after injury).

LACHESIS MUTA

Modalities

< ON WAKING. Morning on rising. AFTER SLEEP. After midnight.

< Before or during MENSES. TOUCH, even of pillow or combing hair.

< *Heat*, SUN. Uncovering head. Coldness or cold, wet weather.

< MOTION, stooping, rising from bed, coughing, heavy stepping, sitting, ascending stairs. Mental exertion.

> By flow: NASAL DISCHARGE, nose bleed, flow of menses.

> Cold or sometimes warm applications. OPEN AIR.

> LYING. After EATING. *External pressure.*Wrapping up the head.

▼ SYMPTOM PROFILE

Psychological

• Talkative, witty, sarcastic. Sad & anxious. Jealousy, SUSPICION.

• Suppression of *sexual or aggressive instincts* with GUILT, fanaticism.

• Effects of emotional strain, broken heart, grief, anger.

Metabolic

• WARM-BLOODED < HEAT. Tendency to hemorrhage.

• Emaciated. Weak. Abuse of alcohol. FLUSHING and heat.

• LEFT-sided problems generally, though headaches often on right.

Women

• MENOPAUSE: flushes, headache, palpitations, hemorrhage.

• Dysmenorrhea, endometriosis. All symptoms > flow of menses.

• Ovarian cysts, inflammation. Fibroids, ovarian or uterine cancer.

Throat: Left-sided sore throat < hot drinks, empty swallowing, *touch*.

▼ DOSAGE

Potency

• The 30th is best. Higher potencies only if symptom profile matches.

Repetition

• Very deep-acting remedy; it can produce a strong healing crisis.

• Allow one dose to finish its action completely. REPEAT RARELY.

▼ CLINICAL CONDITIONS

• Headache • Injury • Migraine • Neuralgia • Spastic paralysis
• Sprains (with bluish swelling of joints) • Wounds, punctures.

LACHNANTES

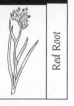

Red Root

▼ KEYNOTES

➤ Neck pain and STIFFNESS. *Torticollis*; drawn to the right.
➤ Migraine headache, with chills < noise, after vomiting, motion.
➤ Icy coldness between shoulder blades.

▼ NECK SYMPTOMS

Pain

• Intense neck pain, *as if dislocated.*
• TEARING pain radiating to shoulder and elbow; may run upwards or down < turning head, bending back or sideways.
• STIFFNESS, spasm; *head drawn to the side* (< right side). Unable to straighten neck due to pain. Pain in sternomastoid muscle.
• Torticollis from neck problem or sore throat. Pains into the jaw.

Associated

• Icy coldness between shoulder blades. CHILLINESS.
• Red blotches on the cheeks; eyes brilliantly clear.
• Burning of palms and soles.
• Bubbling in the heart or chest, rising to the head. With vertigo.

Modalities

< MOTION, turning, on waking, RIGHT side.
> Heat.

▼ HEADACHE SYMPTOMS

• RIGHT-SIDED migraine headache.
• Bursting, splitting pain on right. Dull or tearing pain in forehead.
• Pain into the jaws. CHILLS; alternately hot and cold.
• Expanded sensation on vertex of the head. Extreme *soreness of scalp.*
• Bridge of nose feels pinched. Must keep eyes closed.
< Movement, vomiting. SLIGHTEST NOISE, even walking on carpet.

37 •

LACHNANTES TINCTORIA

▼ LOW BACK SYMPTOMS

- Burning in sacrum and low back.
- TEARING pain into the *buttocks*, knees, toes, with cramps in the legs < lying in bed, walking.
- Legs fall asleep, with tingling and prickling.

▼ SYMPTOM PROFILE

Psychological
- Excitable, TALKATIVE. Bold speech.
- Sadness. Bitter crying spells.
- When dozing off sees images, ghosts, fantasies.

Metabolic
- CHILLY. Shivers and goose bumps.

Digestive
- Rumbling in the intestines. Passing of gas with diarrhea.

Respiratory
- Lachnantes has been used in diphtheria, tuberculosis, pneumonia.

▼ DOSAGE

Potency
- 6, 12, or 30. Lower potencies. Tincture may be applied locally.

Repetition
- May be repeated as needed.

▼ CLINICAL CONDITIONS

- Brachial neuralgia • Cervical arthritis or rheumatism • Cervicalgia (neck pain syndromes) • Facial neuralgia • Low back pain • Migraine headache • Torticollis (Wry neck).

"The white pigs and sheep of Virginia lose their hoofs if they feed on Lachnantes, while the black varieties eat it without inconvenience." — Dr. John H. Clarke from the Dictionary of the Practical Materia Medica, 1900.

LEDUM

Labrador Tea

▼ **KEYNOTES**

➣ Rheumatism, gout < warmth, heat of the bed > COLD bathing.
➣ Arthritis, synovitis of the limbs, travel upward. Nodosities.
➣ Joints SWOLLEN, cold, pale. Bruising. Puncture wounds.

▼ **MUSCULOSKELETAL SYMPTOMS**

Pain

• *Types of pain*: 1. Tearing 2. Pressing 3. Drawing 4. Stitching or sore.
• Extreme tenderness.

Location

• Rheumatism, gout, inflammation of the peripheral joints, including the *shoulders, elbows, hands, hip, knee, ankles, feet,* and *heels*.
• Rheumatism or pains *travel upward*; from the foot, to the knee and up.
• May be cross-lateral arthritis; e.g. left shoulder and right hip.
• *Shoulder*: Stitching pain < on raising the arm, motion.
• *Hands*: Stiff. Drawing pain from hand upwards. Arthritic nodosities.
• *Hip*: Stiff. Stitching pain < standing, walking. B*ubbling, boiling feeling.*
• *Leg*: Drawing in hollow of the knee. Cramps in calves. Heavy limbs.
• *Knee*: Tearing pain. Cracking, swelling, stiffness < walking.
• *Feet*: Ankles sprain easily. Swelling of the feet up to the knee.
  Painful soles, heels feel bruised < walking, stepping.
  Gout of big toe. Itching of feet, ankles < scratching and *heat of the bed*.

Associated

• SWOLLEN, COLD to touch with *pale* joints; or may be HOT joints.
• NODOSITIES, deposits, hard swelling of the joints.
• STIFFNESS of elbow, wrist, fingers, knee, ankle, *foot* > cold.
• CONTRACTION of tendons and muscle, including the hamstrings, calf, heels, hollow of the knee.
• CRACKING in joints, especially the knee.
• *Trembling* (leg, hand) on motion, walking, grasping, sitting, standing.
• Weak joints with easy spraining. Weakness of the limbs. Heaviness.
• Emaciation of the affected area. Heat and burning of the limbs.
• Bruising; mottled or purplish *discolorations*.

38

• •

LEDUM PALUSTRE

Modalities
< HEAT of BED or covers. WARMTH, though chilly. *Slightest pressure.*
< MOTION. WALKING. Stepping, rising up from a seat.
< Standing. SITTING (though often forced to rest by pain, etc.).
< Evening and NIGHT (ankles < the in morning). Wine.
< TOUCH. *Rubbing* (though rubbing relieves hip, knee, or leg pain).
> COLD APPLICATIONS, *ice cold baths* or compresses. REST.

▼ SYMPTOM PROFILE

Psychological
• Aversion to company, to people. Seeks solitude.

Metabolic
• CHILLY but < warmth of the bed. Strong, robust, fleshy. Red face.
• Effects of alcoholism (particularly from whiskey).
• Uricemia and gout. For toxicity of gout medication e.g. Colchicine.
• Eczema and papular eruptions. Antidote to poison ivy.

▼ DOSAGE

Potency
• 3rd to 30th.

Repetition
• *First aid*: Daily doses until bruising and swelling disappear.
• *Arthritis or gout*: Long-acting remedy. Use infrequent or single doses.

▼ CLINICAL CONDITIONS

First Aid
• *Bruising*, ecchymosis. Bruises that remain a long time. *Black eye.*
• Intense soreness after injuries.
• Puncture wounds and bites of insects or animals.
• Retinal or conjunctival hemorrhage.
• Wounds are *cold to the touch, yet > by cold applications.*

Musculoskeletal
• Achilles tendonitis • Arthritis (subacute or chronic phases)
• Arthritis deformans • Back injuries • Cracking of joints • Gout
• Hip disease • Knee synovitis or bursitis (Housemaid's knee)
• Nodosities • Recurrent sprains with swelling, bruising
• Rheumatism • Shoulder rheumatism • Synovitis.

LYCOPODIUM

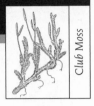

Club Moss

▼ KEYNOTES

➤ Sciatica: Attacks of burning pain < lying on side, rest > walking.
➤ Low back pain < sitting, standing, rising up, morning > urination.
➤ Rheumatism and gout. Chronic digestive problems, bloating.

▼ MUSCULOSKELETAL SYMPTOMS

- SCIATICA: *Burning*, stinging. Pain from hip to foot. Right side.
  Attacks every four days. Limps with pain. Twitches, jerking.
  Cramps in calves, toes.
  < *Lying on painful side, first movement*, sitting, rest, p.m., in bed.
  > Warmth of the bed, WALKING.
- LOW BACK PAIN, extending to the abdomen. Sacrum pain. *Stiffness*.
  Pain in the first lumbar vertebrae at the level of the floating ribs.
  Weakness of back at night.
  < Sitting, standing, night, rising from sitting, stooping, slightest
  motion, a.m. on rising, night, during stool. > *After urination*.
- NECK: Pain shoots to the elbow, arm and hand, only when in bed.
  Stiffness, torticollis with head drawn to the left. Neck tension with
  writing or walking in open air. One side of neck stiff and swollen.
- JOINTS: Rheumatism and nodosities. *Stiffness*, cracking joints.
  Contraction of muscles and tendons.
  Cramps in hands, feet.
  Clumsy, awkward. Restless legs at night.
- HEAD: Headache alternating with joint pains.
  < Afternoon (4-8 p.m.), mental exertion, becoming *warm*.
  > Walking in the open air.
- SPINE: Burning pain between the scapulae.
  Heat and burning along the spine.
- SHOULDER: Tearing pain in the right shoulder < rest > motion.
- HIP: Tearing and stitching < sitting, rising, pressure > walking.

LYCOPODIUM CLAVATUM

Modalities
< First motion, sitting, lying down > Continued motion. WALKING.
< WARM room or air, hot applications > Warmth of bed (sciatica).
< Touch. Cold, DRAFTS. DAMP or living in a damp place.
< Morning, on awakening. 4-8 p.m. After midnight.
< Exertion. RIGHT SIDE.
> Cool OPEN AIR, uncovering head, cold applications. Dry weather.

▼ SYMPTOM PROFILE

Psychological
• Oversensitive and intellectual. Easily angered, impatient.
• Domineering, fault-finding, pretentious. Self-centered, stingy.
• Lack of confidence. Cowardly. Fear of failure, disease, being alone.
• Gradual or progressive loss of mental and physical powers.

Metabolic
• Intellectually strong, physically weak. Thin, emaciated.
• Craves fresh, open air < warm room or air, though CHILLY.
• < 4-8 p.m. Right side or from right to left side. Desires sweets.
• Tendency to high uric acid; gout and deposits of tophi.

Digestive
• Chronic weak digestion. Increased appetite, yet easily full.
• Sour dyspepsia. Spastic constipation.

▼ DOSAGE

Potency
• Up to the 200th potency in rheumatic complaints.

Repetition
• A gradual and deep-acting remedy. Infrequent repetitions needed.

▼ CLINICAL CONDITIONS

• Brachial neuralgia • Gout • Headache • Heel pain • Hip joint disease
• Knee rheumatism (stiffness) • Low back pain • Rheumatism
• Sciatica • Shoulder • Torticollis.

NAT MUR

NaCl
Common Salt

▼ KEYNOTES

➤ MIGRAINE: Aura of flashing light, hammering pain < heat, daytime.
➤ Low back pain, weakness < stooping > pressure, *lying on hard surface.*
➤ Suppressed grief < sympathy. Weak, thirsty, craves fresh air.

▼ HEADACHE SYMPTOMS

Pain

• Onset of *blindness* or ZIGZAGS of light. Numbness, tingling of face.
• Throbbing, bursting, HAMMERING inside. Stitching, shooting.

Location

• Forehead, vertex (as from a blow). *One-sided*, on alternating sides.

Associated

• Pale. *Nausea and watery vomiting.* FAINTNESS. Violent jerks in head.
• DRY MOUTH and *thirst.* Pain draws eyes together.
• *Causes:* Emotions (depression, anger, suppressed tears, etc.), eye-strain, anemia, sinusitis, fluid loss, fasting, pressure of a hat.

Modalities

< On rising, 10 a.m., sunrise to sunset, menses. ALTERNATE DAYS.
< HEAT of sun, summer, *warm room*, moist heat. Seashore.
< Moving head or eyes, bright light, noise, reading, coughing.
< Sympathy or consolation, talking, any mental exertion.
> *Open air*, cool bathing. Pressure (on eyes). Rest. Fasting. Sweating.

▼ LOW BACK SYMPTOMS

• Beaten, bruised, LAME, as if broken. Cutting, pulsating pains.
• Sharp stitches horizontally across the back < a.m., at night.
• *Weakness*, AS IF PARALYZED, *numbness* < morning. Chills in the back.
• Sensitive spine, between vertebrae < touch, pressure.

Modalities

< Prolonged STOOPING, SITTING, *rising from sitting*, or straightening.
< MORNING on rising. After eating. After stool.
< Lying (left side). Sitting. Before sleep. Deep breath, coughing.
> Pressure or LYING ON A HARD SURFACE, lying on the back.
> Supporting the spine, leaning on something. *Frequent turning in bed.*

• •

NATRUM MURIATICUM

▼ **Other Locations & Symptoms**

- STIFFNESS, rigidity of muscles and joints. Arthritic swelling.
- Cracking of joints. *Restless* limbs. Limbs and spine feel WEAK.
- Cramps, twitching, trembling, and weakness.
- *Neck* thin and emaciated. Stitches in neck and occiput. Stiffness.
- *Thoracic:* Tearing pain between scapulae < sitting, lying > deep breath, walking. Weak, fatigued feeling. Pain, as if it would break.
- *Extremities:* Contraction of hamstrings. Hands and feet go to sleep; tingling and numbness. Hip rheumatism. Ankles sprain easily. Cold feeling in joints, as if water trickling over them.

▼ **Symptom Profile**

Psychological

- DEPRESSED, weepy, hopeless. *Emotional trauma*, but suppressed.
- Feels forsaken, alone, yet DESIRES SOLITUDE and *hates sympathy.*
- Responsible, caring, yet cautious. Cannot let go of past hurts.

Metabolic

- Chilly but worse from heat or the sun. *Craves fresh air.*
- Anemia, emaciation. Thin, malnourished. Thirsty, craves salt.
- Weakness. Hyperthyroid, low adrenal function. Amenorrhea.

Respiratory

- Common cold. Allergy and hay fever. Watery discharge.

Skin

- Greasy, oily skin. Herpes simplex. Hives.

Digestive

- Constipation, contraction of the anus. Dry hard stools.

▼ **Dosage**

Potency

- Lowest to highest potencies, depending on the correspondence to symptoms and the constitutional typology. Generally 6th to 30th.

Repetition

- Daily doses of low potencies until a response, or a single high dose.

▼ **Clinical Conditions**

- Hip disease (early stages) • Housemaid's knee • Low back pain
- Migraine headache • Neck pain • Rheumatism • Shoulder bursitis.

NAT SULPH

Na$_2$SO$_4$

Sodium Sulphate

▼ KEYNOTES

➤ Joint and muscular rheumatism. Hip or knee disease. Sciatica.
➤ Head injury resulting in epilepsy, mental changes, or depression.
➤ < DAMPNESS, REST, lying, rising up, touch > Motion, rubbing.

▼ MUSCULOSKELETAL SYMPTOMS

Pain
• Tearing, pressing, drawing, burning pains. Piercing pains.

Location
• *Hip Joint*: Sudden stitching, extends to the knee, prevents walking.
  < LEFT side, resting, rising up from a seat, sitting, stooping, turning
  in bed, night. Moves constantly to relieve the pain.
• *Knees*: STIFFNESS, cracking. Contraction of muscles and tendons in
  hollow of the knee. Weakness of thigh, knee, leg, ankle. Burning.
• Contraction of calf muscles on walking, stepping. Extends to knee.
• *Neck*: Pain extends to head, clavicle < turning, stretching, yawning.
• *Low Back and Sacrum*: Pain after injury < REST > motion, rubbing,
  lying on the right side. Painful in bed, better after rising.
• *Sciatica*: < Rising up from sitting, turning in bed, LYING too long in
  one position, stooping. No position relieves.
• *Head*: Motion or looseness in the head < stooping.
• *Thorax*: Pain between the shoulder blades.
• *Hand*: Pain on grasping anything.
• *Feet*: Sharp stitches, throbbing in the heels when sitting or standing.

Trauma
• Chief remedy for effects of HEAD INJURY including convulsions,
  depression, irritability, alterations in consciousness, confusion,
  headache with light sensitivity and salivation. Spinal injury.

Modalities
< DAMP: weather, rooms, basements, night air, fog, bathing, getting
  wet, watery foods, living near water, at the seashore, in the tropics,
  warm wet weather. Spring. Wind. Change of weather, i.e. dry to wet.

41

NATRUM SULPHURICUM

< REST (though some pains < motion). TOUCH, pressure.
< LYING down, *lying on the left side* (hip, wrist, knee, ankle, etc.).
< Morning, on waking, late evening, 4-5 p.m. From lifting.
> MOTION, change of position, walking, stretching. Sitting up.
> RUBBING the limb. Dry weather. Dry heat. OPEN AIR. Midday.

Associated
• RESTLESS on account of the pain. Stiffness of the limbs on motion.
• Compressive feeling in the joints (leg, wrist, ankle, elbow).

▼ SYMPTOM PROFILE

Psychological
• DEPRESSION. *Suicidal impulse* < MUSIC, mental exertion.
• Many vivid, fantastic, and frightening dreams. Wakes frequently.

Metabolic
• CHILLY. Sensitive to pain, cold. Water retention.

Respiratory
• ASTHMA < damp conditions. Diarrhea with each attack.

Abdomen
• DIARRHEA with rumbling, gurgling. Sudden gushing, noisy stools in the morning after rising. HEPATITIS. Gallstones. Jaundice.

Skin
• Eruptions every spring. Red WARTS. Eczema. Yellow discharges.

▼ DOSAGE

Potency
• Useful from the lowest to the highest potencies.

Repetition
• Low potency (6x) repeated often. Otherwise occasional doses.

▼ CLINICAL CONDITIONS

• Coccyx pain • Gout • Head injury (epilepsy, concussion, headache)
• Heel pain • HIP JOINT DISEASE • Knee rheumatism
• Low back pain (after injury)• Neck pain • Sciatica.

NUX VOMICA

Poison Nut

▼ KEYNOTES

➤ Tension and spasm + Weakness and paralysis.

➤ < COLD — TOUCH — MOTION, A.M., dry > WARMTH, wet.

➤ IRRITABLE, driven. Overindulgence in stimulants. Constipation.

▼ MUSCULOSKELETAL SYMPTOMS

Headache

• Occiput or forehead, above eye. Pressing, stitching, sore, bruised. < A.M., on waking, COLD, eating, light, noise > evening, rising, lying, pressure, WARMTH, wrapping head warmly, eating.

• Head feels expanded; larger than the body. Vertigo and faintness.

• Scalp sore, internal soreness. Nausea, vomiting.

Associated

• *Vertigo & FAINTNESS.* Photophobia. *Urging to stool.*

• *Causes:* Stimulants, *coffee,* alcohol, tobacco, overeating, rich foods, *loss of sleep,* sun, *cold air* or winds, common cold, mental strain or overwork, ANGER.

Back pain

• LUMBAR or sacral pain: *Bruised,* but may be sharp, tearing, spasmodic, drawing, constrictive, burning, lame. Feels "as if broken." Electric pains. *Drives him out of bed at 4 a.m.* Crawling along the spine. *Must sit up in order to turn over* when lying. Worse stooping, turning. Radiates to the hips. Sudden stitches on turning. Stiffness.

• NECK: Cramping, tearing into shoulder. Heavy, STIFF. Left torticollis.

• THORAX: Pain, tension or burning between the scapulae.

Extremities

• DRAWING, darting, stitching pains. Affects large joints & muscles.

• SPASM, tension, *contraction of muscles and tendons* < yawning.

• Twitches and tremblings. HEAVY, lethargic limbs. NUMBNESS.

• WEAK or paralyzed limbs, arms, or legs (or both) in the morning.

• *Knee:* Inflammation, swelling. Cramps in calves. Cracking of joints. Sensation in hollow of knee as if the tendons were shortened.

• *Sciatica:* radiating to the back of the knee < lifting or trying to stand.

42

NUX VOMICA

Modalities

< COLD, open air, dry cold, uncovering. MOTION. Lying on the back.
< TOUCH, tight clothing. Noise, odors, light. Eating
< Early *morning*: 3-4 a.m., on waking and also < evening (pains).
< Right side. Mental exertion or overstrain. Coffee, alcohol, drugs.
> WRAPPING WARMLY, *hot applications*. PRESSURE. *Damp, wet*.
> *Napping*, rest, sitting, lying on the left or painless side.
> *Evening* (headache). Loosening clothing.

▼ **SYMPTOM PROFILE**

Psychological

• DRIVEN. Ambitious, overachiever, workaholic. Fastidious.
• IRRITABLE, quarrelsome, malicious, impatient. *Critical, fault-finding*.
• TENSE. Cramped, blocked, uptight. *Can't relax*. Sullen and silent.
• Business worries and stress. Sedentary lifestyle. Burn-out.

Metabolic

• CHILLY. *Cold limbs, hands, and feet*. Faintness. Muscular tension.
• *Hypersensitive* to PAIN, to noise, light, odors, touch.
• Craving and overindulgence in stimulants, food, late nights.
• ANTIDOTE to many types of drugs, stimulants, coffee, etc.

Digestive: Indigestion. Ulcers. Spastic constipation with urging.

Sleep: *Insomnia*. Wakes 3-4 a.m, with busy mind. Unrefreshed sleep.

▼ **DOSAGE**

Potency

• 6th to 30 for headache or low back pain. High potencies for constitutional types. Take before bedtime, not after meals or in the a.m.

Repetition:

• A short-acting remedy, though not to be repeated too frequently.
• One to three times daily in acutes. Single doses of higher potency.

▼ **CLINICAL CONDITIONS**

• Brachial neuralgia • Headache • Low back pain • Lumbar neuralgia
• Pain sensitivity • Sciatica • Spasms • Spastic paralysis
• Sprain of a single part, muscle or tendon • Torticollis • Trauma.

PHYTOLACCA

Poke Root

▼ KEYNOTES

➤ Fibrous inflammation with stiffness. Shifting, shooting pains.

➤ 1. Soreness 2. Restlessness 3. Weakness. Swollen, hot joints.

➤ < Damp — Cold — Motion, rising up > Warmth, dry, rest.

▼ MUSCULOSKELETAL SYMPTOMS

Pain

• SORENESS ALL OVER, aching. Shock-like, electric shooting pains.

• Stitching, pressing pains, *changing rapidly. Shoot up and down.*

• Abrupt onset and cessation of pains. Onset after tonsillitis.

Location

• Acts on *fibrous sheaths* of bone (periosteum), muscle, nerves, fascia, tendinous attachments. *Outer aspect of limbs.* Fibrositis, exostoses.

• NECK: *Stiffness* < morning. Pain, running down the spine or extending to the occiput. Aching in scapulae. Intercostal rheumatism.

• LOW BACK: Constant aching pain, heaviness in lumbar spine and sacrum. Stiff every a.m. LBP, sciatica, or hip joint disease with pain radiating from the sacrum along *lateral thighs* to the knees and toes.

• UPPER LIMBS: Right arm numb and fuzzy. Right shoulder stiff with shooting pain. Cannot raise the arms. *Pain below the knees and elbows.*

• LOWER LIMBS: Tight hamstrings. Knotted cramps come and go.

• Heels ache > elevating feet or lying. Weak and heavy. Aching tibia.

• BONE PAINS at night or from damp and cold.

Associated

• RESTLESS yet < motion. Muscular SORENESS.

• *Stiffness* of the whole body, lameness. Debility after the pain.

• WEAKNESS, lassitude. Groans with each movement.

• Swelling, redness, HEAT of the joints. Nodosities.

• Contraction of muscles and tendons of the legs, hamstrings.

• Inflammation stays in one joint for hours, then goes to another.

Modalities

< DAMP, COLD, damp climate, rain, open air. *Pressure.*

43

PHYTOLACCA DECANDRA

< MOTION, rising, walking. Night (bones, sciatica), *morning* (joints).
< Change of weather. Electrical changes. Right side. Warmth (hip).
> WARMTH. Dry weather. Resting, *lying down* on abdomen. Daytime.

▼ SYMPTOM PROFILE

Psychological
- *Indifference*, loathing and weariness of life. DEPRESSION, gloom and melancholy < rainy weather. Loss of personal delicacy.

Metabolic
- WEAK, great exhaustion, with the wish to lie down. Faint on rising.
- *Glandular* enlargements and inflammation. Swollen neck glands.
- Cold hands and feet.
- Phytolacca has anti-tumor, anti-cancer effects.
- Acts on adhesions and scar tissue.

Breasts
- Acute MASTITIS < during breast-feeding. Mammary tumors, cancer.
- Pain radiates from the nipple to the back, chest, or whole body.

Throat
- Sore throat, TONSILLITIS. Throat dark red or bluish.
- Hot ball or sticking sensation. Painful swallowing.

▼ DOSAGE

Potency
- 6, 12, or 30 (x or c). Low potencies for advanced joint changes.

Repetition
- In acute cases, three or more times daily. In chronic cases, 6c three times daily for several weeks, or single doses of the 30th.

▼ CLINICAL CONDITIONS

- Arthritis • Bursitis • Cervical pain, arthritis • Exostoses • Fasciitis
- Fibromyalgia • Gout • Heel inflammation • Hip joint disease
- Joint contracture • Knee rheumatism • Low back pain • Myositis
- Periosteal injury or disease • Rheumatism (subacute and chronic)
- Scar tissue • Sciatica • Shoulder-arm-hand syndrome • Tendonitis
- TMJ problems • Torticollis.

PULSATILLA

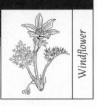

Windflower

▼ KEYNOTES

➣ JOINT INFLAMMATION; tearing, stinging pains. Episodic pain.
➣ Shifting location. Affects the large joints with swelling, redness.
➣ < Heat > Cold bathing. < Rest, first motion > Continued motion.

▼ MUSCULOSKELETAL SYMPTOMS

Pain
• Shifting, CHANGING locations and quality of pain.
• TEARING, *stinging*, sharp, intense. Episodes or paroxysms of pain.
• Appear suddenly, build up, cease gradually or *let up with a snap*.

Location
• Erratic, *wandering pains*, from joint to joint, but usually one-sided.
• Affects large joints: Shoulders, wrists, hips, *knees*, ankles.
• SPINE: Whole back, painfully *stiff as a board*. Sticking pains.
• NECK: Pain in the muscles (left) as from lying in a wrong position. Sticking or shooting pain in nape of the neck. Swelling of the area.
• THORAX: Interscapular pain < inspiration. Thoracic scoliosis.
• LOW BACK or sacrum pain, as if sprained. *Constriction as from a tight band* < after sitting, long stooping, morning. Must move, but in low back pain or sciatica, motion does not relieve!

Associated
• RESTLESS. Chilly with the pain, yet < heat. *As if cold water on her back*.
• *Redness* and SWELLING (mild to severe). Heaviness, numbness.
• From suppressed sweat, menses, chilling, getting wet, WET FEET.
• *Numbness of parts lain on*. Cracking, trembling, cramping. Stiffness.

Modalities
< WARMTH in any form (weather, room, air, clothes, bed). Storms.
< *Evening*. Every other night. During menses. Jarring.
< REST and *initial motion*. Rising up from sitting (low back pain).
< Lying on one side (left). Letting the limbs hang down. Pressure.
> *Open air*, fresh air. Cold, COLD APPLICATIONS.
> *Gentle* or CONTINUED MOTION, walking. Lying on the painful side.

PULSATILLA NIGRICANS

▼ **SYMPTOM PROFILE**

Psychological
- Mild, timid, gentle, *sweet*, affectionate, shy or PASSIVE.
- WEEPY. Likes sympathy. Broken heart, loneliness. Whining.
- Unfulfilled love. Better after a good cry. Changeable moods.

Metabolic
- WARM, and worse with warmth. CRAVES FRESH, OPEN AIR.
- Fair complexion and hair. Fleshy or overweight.
- Anemia. Thirstlessness. Venous problems, varicose veins.
- Complaints that began at puberty, during pregnancy, or menses.
- < Eating rich food, pork. Problems from getting wet or suppressing natural discharges (sweat, menses, tears, etc.).

Eye, Nose, Throat
- OTITIS MEDIA. Styes, mucus discharge. Yellow, thick, bland discharges from the eye, nose, throat, sinuses, etc.

Digestive
- Indigestion, heartburn, and dyspepsia. Averse to and < fats, rich foods, pork. Heavy, undigested feeling. Distention.

Women
- Hormonal disturbances; amenorrhea or scanty menses.
- PMS with irritability and tender breasts. Dysmenorrhea.

▼ **DOSAGE**

Potency
- 6th to 30th in joint complaints. Higher doses if constitutional type.

Repetition
- Repeated doses of low potencies or single dose of high.

▼ **CLINICAL CONDITIONS**

- Arthritis • Brachial neuralgia • Bursitis • Foot (heel) pain, swelling
- Gout • Headache • Knee bursitis (Housemaid's knee)
- Low back pain • Neuralgia • Polyarthritis • Rheumatism
- Sciatica • Shoulder bursitis • Synovitis (of large joints)
- Tennis elbow • Wrist tendonitis.

RANUNCULUS

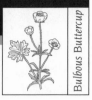

Bulbous Buttercup

▼ **KEYNOTES**

➤ *Thoracic pain*, myalgia, neuralgia with stitching pains, tenderness.
➤ Pain from SITTING STOOPED OVER, fine work, typing, writing.
➤ < *Motion*, touch, cold, damp, change of weather or temperature.

▼ **MUSCULOSKELETAL SYMPTOMS**

Pain
• Sharp, stitching, shooting. Bruised soreness. Intense episodes.

Location
• Affects muscle and nerve tissue in general; neuralgia and myalgia.
• THORACIC SPINE. *Between the shoulder blades*, along the ribs, along the *left margin or* lower angle of the scapula.
• *Low back:* Sore, bruised, in upper lumbars. Stitching, shooting to front.
• Burning in small spots around the ribs, spine, and scapulae.

Causes
• Muscular pain and spasm in the back and hands from typing, writing, fine work, overwork. From excessive or *prolonged bending over*.
• Office workers who sit hunched over a table, etc.
• Effects of anger, injuries. After getting chilled.

Associated
• Muscles sore, TENDER to the touch, and stiff from overuse.
• Acute intercostal neuralgia. Costal cartilages tender, sore.
• Irritable, chilly. Restless.
• Weakness and lassitude felt in the limbs.

Modalities
< MOTION, *change of position*, turning, moving arms, writing, breathing in deeply, sitting or bending forward, walking, *lying*.
< COLD air, DAMP air, fresh or open air. DRAFTS. Stormy weather.
< *Changes of weather or temperature* (warm to cold or dry to wet).
< TOUCH. Pressure. Left side.
< Alcohol. EVENING or early morning on waking.
> Warm applications, warm weather. Drawing up the limbs.

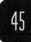

45 •

RANUNCULUS BULBOSUS

▼ Symptom Profile

Psychological
- IRRITABLE, quarrelsome, fits of temper. *Easily offended.*
- Confused, difficult concentration. Fear of ghosts.

Metabolic
- Very CHILLY. Lassitude. Bruised feeling all over.
- ALCOHOLISM (an important remedy).
- Delirium tremens, liver disease, and ascites.

Respiratory
- Pleurisy. Pleuritic adhesions. Acute colds.

Skin
- Herpes zoster (shingles). Vesicular eruptions with pricking or burning pains and itching < on the thorax, hands, above the eyes.

▼ Dosage

Potency
- 3rd to 30th potency. Additionally, a low potency, mixed with water, may be rubbed onto the heels in chronic sciatica.

Repetition
- A short-acting remedy.
- Repeated doses may be used until improvement is noted.

▼ Clinical Conditions

- Brachial neuralgia • Facial neuralgia over right eye < lying > walking and standing (all other symptoms < motion) • Fibromyalgia
- INTERCOSTAL NEURALGIA • Low back pain • Muscular strain
- Myalgia • Myositis • Pleurodynia • Rheumatism • Rib pain after respiratory illness • Sciatica (chronic; not > lying down)
- THORACIC NEURALGIA OR MYALGIA • Thoracic subluxations
- Writer's cramp.

RHODODENDRON

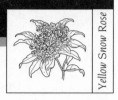

Yellow Snow Rose

▼ KEYNOTES

➤ Rheumatism with wandering, tearing, deep-seated pains.
➤ Small joints. Pain in small spots. Forearms, lower legs.
➤ < BEFORE and during a STORM. Cold, damp. Rest, a.m. > Motion.

▼ MUSCULOSKELETAL SYMPTOMS

Pain
• DEEP PAIN, felt in the bone and periosteum. Joints "as if strained."
• *Tearing*, zigzag, boring pain, with weakening effects.
• Neuralgic, erratic, changeable pains. PAIN IN SMALL SPOTS.

Location
• WANDERING PAINS, changeable location, joint to joint.
• Chronic inflammation of connective tissue, joints, tendons at their site of attachment, muscle, nerve. Bone and periosteum.
• Affinity to the small joints (fingers and toes), forearm, lower limbs.
• NECK: Stiffness. Tearing pain, flying down the back and elsewhere.
• LOW BACK: Aching pain < sitting, damp, morning, stooping.
• SHOULDER: Weakness, tearing pain, formication in the forearms.
• WRIST: Feels sprained. *Heel pain.* Podagra (gout of the big toe).

Associated
• Arthritic NODOSITIES, chalky deposits.
• Swelling. Bursitis, neuralgia. RED swelling of joints.
• Weakness felt during rest • Must *sleep with the legs crossed.*

Modalities
< BEFORE a STORM, during a storm, weather changes, *cold, damp,* cloudy, getting wet. *Windy weather.* Change of seasons, spring, fall.
< Barometric changes and *electrical changes.* In hot weather!
< NIGHT, just before MORNING. *Wine.* Right side (or left then right).
< REST (like Rhus tox but little stiffness). Sitting too long, etc.
> *After the storm breaks.* Being in the sun, sunshine.
> *Dry heat.* Wrapping up warmly.
> MOTION, continued motion or walking.

RHODODENDRON CHRYSANTHUM

▼ SYMPTOM PROFILE

Psychological
- NERVOUS BEFORE STORMS. *Fear of thunder.* Anxiety, fear of touch.
- Confused, forgetful in speaking, writing. Vanishing of thoughts.
- Morose, gloomy, indifferent.

Metabolic
- Pains reappear before a storm, causing anxiety.
- Cold feet even in warm room or bed. Hands warm in cold weather.
- Feet feel like there is a weight on them, feel as if asleep.
- *Cannot sleep unless the legs are crossed.*

Head
- Rheumatic headache < in bed > motion.
- Facial or dental neuralgia or TMJ pain < damp, windy weather, before storm > eating.
- Vertigo < lying in bed > motion. Tinnitus aurium.

Male
- Orchitis: Acute or chronic testicular swelling and inflammation.

▼ DOSAGE

Potency
- Up to the 30th or 200th. Best given in the evening.

Repetition
- Single doses repeated when symptoms indicate.

▼ CLINICAL CONDITIONS

Nerves
- Brachial neuralgia • Dental neuralgia • Facial neuralgia • Sciatica.

Joints
- Achilles tendonitis • Arthritis of small joints • Bursitis • Gout
- Heel pain • Jaw pain > motion • Low back pain • Neck pain
- Nodosities of finger joints • Rheumatism • Rheumatoid arthritis
- Shoulder disorders • Sprains • Tendonitis • Torticollis • Wrist pain.

RHUS TOX

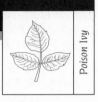

Poison Ivy

▼ KEYNOTES

➤ Acute sprains or chronic arthritis, neuralgia. RESTLESS and STIFF.

➤ < DAMP, cold, weather changes > Warmth, hot wraps.

➤ < INITIAL MOTION, after rest > Limbering up < Prolonged motion.

▼ MUSCULOSKELETAL SYMPTOMS

NOTE: As one of the most important joint remedies, Rhus has local symptoms that can be extremely detailed, varied, and confusing. The main *modalities* and *characteristics* should be kept in mind.

Pain

• TEARING, DRAWING, *burning*, stitching, shooting pains.

• Bruised soreness. As if sprained or beaten.

Causes

• DAMP environment. Getting soaked or getting the feet wet.

• CHILLING after overheating or sweating.

• Effects of strains and sprains, over-exertion, surgery.

• The above may have occurred years before onset of the condition.

Locations

• Affinity to connective or fibrous tissue, especially ligaments; Rhus may be useful and effective for literally any joint in the body.

• Chronic joint inflammation at the site of sprains.

• Pains spread over a large area. Left upper and right lower joints.

• HEADACHE from neck rheumatism < bending the head back.

• NECK: Stiffness. Sprained pain from nape to between the scapulae.

• THORAX: Painful tension between the shoulder blades. Curvature of the thoracic spine (scoliosis or kyphosis).

• LOW BACK: Aching, stiff < sitting, resting > pressure, *lying on a hard surface*, walking, bending back. Heaviness, pressure, as if beaten. Back strain. Sudden "crick," violent pain from lifting.

• SCIATICA: Pain down back of the thighs or shooting into the legs. Legs feel dead, wooden. Cramps in calves. After excess exertion.

• SACRUM and coccyx pain with aching into the thighs.

RHUS TOXICODENDRON

- SHOULDER: Tearing, burning pains. Sprained shoulder.
- ARMS: Tearing pain, extending to fingers < rest. Trembling limbs.
- HANDS: Swelling of fingertips. Crawling or tingling sensations. Rheumatism. Hot swelling < evening, wet weather.
- ELBOWS: Pain, epicondylitis (tennis elbow) > motion, warmth.
- WRISTS: Rheumatism, sprains. Swollen, stiff, *pain from side to side*.
- HIP: Pain < ascending or rising from sitting. Pain *at every step*.
- KNEE: Stiffness, heaviness, tension, as if the tendons were too short. Patellar pain. Burning pain, swelling. Pain shooting into leg.
- ANKLE, knee, or foot sprains or rheumatism < sitting > motion.
- FEET: Swelling of the feet at night. Pain in the arches, heels.

Associated
- STIFFNESS after rest, morning, or on first motion.
- Inflamed joints are red, shiny, and swollen. Cracking of joints.
- Extreme RESTLESSNESS, can't rest in any position.
- Need to stretch or move which relieves the pain.
- WEAKNESS. Paralysis, trembling, muscular twitching. These symptoms occur or are < after overwork or exposure to damp or cold.
- *Numbness*, tingling, prickling, or formication (crawling) in the fingers or toes. Limbs fall asleep easily.
- HEAVINESS in the limbs, neck, low back, sacrum. *Lameness*.
- Areas of bony protuberances painful.

Modalities
< ON INITIAL MOTION, *after rest*, or after excess motion or activity.
< Flexing the limb. Lying on the part causes pain (hip, low back).
< DAMP, getting wet, RAIN, *onset of a storm*, cloudy or foggy weather.
< COLD: open air, drafts, air-conditioned environment, uncovering.
< Night. AFTER MIDNIGHT. Evening. Twilight.
< Right side or left to right. Lying on either side > lying on the back.
> CONTINUED MOTION or limbering (like a "rusty gate"), walking.
> *Stretching*, change of position. Lying on a hard surface.
> WARMTH, warm weather, hot bath, wrapping up. Dry weather.
> Warming up from exercise. Rubbing.

RHUS TOXICODENDRON

▼ SYMPTOM PROFILE

Psychological

- FEAR of misfortune, of the future, *of business or financial failure.*
- Fear of being harmed, on guard < twilight and *night.*
- Mentally stiff, with fixed ideas. Withholds feelings. *Superstitious.*
- DEPRESSED. *Weeping;* wants to be alone to cry. Suicidal despair.
- Dwells on unpleasant thoughts or past events.
- RESTLESS anxiety. Anxiety when sitting bent!
- Dreams of roaming the fields, of great physical exertion.

Metabolic

- Easily chilled. Desires milk, aversion to alcohol.
- Triangular red tip of the tongue.
- Remedy for rheumatic fever, flu, typhoid fever, dysentery.

Skin

- Cellulitis, erysipelas. Vesicular or herpetic eruptions. Herpes zoster (shingles). Chickenpox, herpes simplex (cold sores), acne.

Eye

- Inflammation and cellulitis. Iritis or paralysis from cold or damp.

▼ DOSAGE

Potency

- 6, 12, 30 or higher potencies. 200 and higher very effective.

Repetition

- Repeated doses of low potency or single doses of high potency.

▼ CLINICAL CONDITIONS

- Arthritis (acute and chronic) • Brachial neuralgia • Bursitis
- Coxalgia • Dislocation • Fibromyalgia • Hip arthritis
- Knee rheumatism • Low back pain • Neck sprains • Neuralgia
- Osteo-arthritis • Rheumatism • Sciatica • Shoulder bursitis
- Spinal curvature (thorax) • Sprained ligaments • Strains
- Tendon rupture • Tendonitis • Tennis elbow
- TMJ problems (cracking and pain) • Torticollis • Ulnar neuritis
- Weak, lame joints after injury (wrist, ankle) • Wrist sprain, arthritis.

"Rusty gate," better from gradual limbering

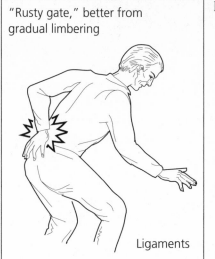

Ligaments

RHUS TOX

• Stiff, restless, sore.
• Tearing pain.

Worse from:
Initial motion, after rest.
Excess activity, overexertion.
Damp, stormy weather.
Cold air, drafts. Cold water.
Night. Twilight.

Better from:
Limbering up.
Stretching, position change.
Heat. Warm, dry weather.

RUTA

• Bruised soreness.
• Weak joints, lameness.
• Restless, weariness.

Worse from:
First motion, exertion.
Sitting, standing.
Lying (except backache).
Stooping, stretching.
Cold, damp. Touch.
Morning, night.

Better from:
Gentle motion. Walking.
Lying flat (backache).
Pressure (backache).
Warmth, dry. rubbing.

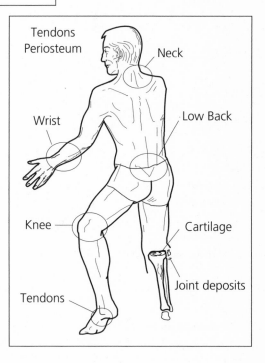

Tendons
Periosteum

Neck

Wrist

Low Back

Knee

Cartilage

Joint deposits

Tendons

RUTA

Garden Rue

▼ KEYNOTES

➤ Joint, tendon, or cartilage injury, DAMAGE or WEAKNESS.
➤ Affinity to wrist, knee, ankles, spine, with nodosities or deposits.
➤ LOW BACK PAIN with restlessness > lying, walking < sitting, cold.

▼ MUSCULOSKELETAL SYMPTOMS

Pain
- BRUISED pain. ACHING SORENESS; locally or of the whole body.
- Part feels "as if broken," as if beaten. Spinal pain as from a fall.

Location
- Tendons, cartilage, periosteum, bone. Sites of tendon insertion.
- SPINE: *Low back pain.* Coccyx: bruised pain. Thoracic scoliosis. Pain after spinal manipulation. Tendency to recurrent subluxations.
- NECK: Cervical arthritis. Neck strains. Stiff neck/torticollis.
- SCIATICA: Deep bone pain, after injury < first motion, sitting or lying, damp or cold, cold applications > walking, motion, rising.
- SHOULDER: Frozen shoulder. Chronic tendonitis or bursitis.
- WRIST: Carpal tunnel syndrome, *sprains, ganglia*, tendonitis, cramp.
- ELBOW: Epicondylitis, i.e., tennis elbow. Tingling in hands.
- KNEE: Sprains, tendonitis, cartilage tears, Baker's cyst, bursitis (Housemaid's knee), Osgood-Schlatter. HIP: Hip joint disease. *Weakness of lower limbs.* Knees give way < on stairs or on rising.
- ANKLE: Weak ankles, tendon nodules. Achilles tendonitis.
- FEET: Sore heels and feet < stepping. Plantar fasciitis.

Associated
- Effects of old fractures, sprains, bruises, lifting. *Repetitive strain.*
- RESTLESSNESS, constant change of position due to soreness.
- DEPOSITS, nodes in tendons, joints, or periosteum after injury.
- WEAK JOINTS: Weak low back < after sitting, difficulty in rising.
- Intense *weariness*, heaviness in the limbs after sitting.
- LAMENESS of the wrist, ankle, or other joints after a strain.
- Stiffness of the wrist, hand, ankle. *Part lain on* becomes sore.

48

RUTA GRAVEOLENS

• Contraction of muscles, tendons: hamstrings, feet, fingers, toes.
• Cracking (crepitus) in joints. Chills in the spine.

Modalities

< SITTING, standing. LYING. *Lying on the painful side.* Stooping, stretching, stepping hard, turning in bed, bending, descending.
< FIRST MOTION, exertion. Averse to motion.
< *Cold* (air, wind, weather). Damp. Cold applications.
< TOUCH. Pressure against a hard edge.
< EVENING. Morning on rising (backache). Night (sciatica).
> CONTINUED MOTION. Walking (except leg pain). Gentle motion.
> LYING FLAT ON THE BACK (backache).
> PRESSURE (backache, sciatica). Daytime. *Warmth*, dry. Rubbing.

▼ **SYMPTOM PROFILE**

Psychological

• ANXIETY; restless and nervous. Many phobias and fears.
• *Fear of death.* Anxiety with sudden stitching spinal pain.
• Despairing mood with joint complaints. Depression in the evening.
• Dissatisfaction with oneself and others. Suspicious.

Metabolic

• Lassitude, weakness, extreme fatigue. < COLD, damp.
• *Starts from sleep with slightest touch.* Vivid, confused dreams. Yawning.

Eyes: EYESTRAIN; soreness, burning, weakness of accommodation.

▼ **DOSAGE**

Potency & Repetition

• 3rd to 200th. Can be repeated frequently.

▼ **CLINICAL CONDITIONS**

• Arthritis • Bone or periosteal injury or inflammation • Bursitis
• Cartilage injury • Dislocations • Fibromyalgia • Fracture (slow healing) • Headache (from eyestrain or neck) • Muscular strain
• Neuralgia (chronic) • Nodes in palms • Nodules in tendons or tissue after injury or bruise • Repetitive strain disorders
• Rheumatism • Sciatica • Spinal curvature • Spinal injury • Sprains
• Trauma • Tendonitis • Weak joints or ligaments.

SANGUINARIA

Blood Root

▼ KEYNOTES

➣ Migraine: RIGHT occiput to temple & EYE with flushed cheeks.
➣ < Daytime, every 7th day, odors > VOMITING, pressure, lying.
➣ Right-sided BURSITIS of the shoulder < raising arm, night.

▼ HEADACHE SYMPTOMS

Pain
• BURSTING, pulsating, *pressing*, boring, or electric-like pains.
• Eye pain PRESSES OUTWARD. ②

Location
• Occiput or trapezius ① radiating to RIGHT EYE, temple, forehead.

Associated
• FLUSHING, burning, and heat. *Circumscribed redness of cheeks.* ③
• Distended temporal veins. Burning palms & soles.
• VOMITING WHICH RELIEVES ④. Vomiting of bile, belching of gas.

Modalities
< Motion, touch, jar, noise, light, ODORS. Cold and damp.
< Every SEVENTH DAY, or on a day of rest. RIGHT side.
< *With the sun*: Starts in a.m., is worst at noon, and lessens till sunset.
< Nasal blockage, SUN, going without food. *Lying with the head low.*
> VOMITING (though it is exhausting). Release of gas or *urination*.
> LYING and REST, lying on the back, *sleep*, DARK, QUIET.
> Hard pressure; *burrowing the head into the pillow.* Cool air.

▼ SHOULDER SYMPTOMS

• RIGHT shoulder, deltoid pain ⑤. Sharp, cutting pain with stiffness.
• Pain radiates into neck, head, or down to hand; in ball of thumb. ⑥
• Cannot move the arm without help; hangs at the side.
• Pain disappears on being touched and appears in some other area.
< MOTION. Turning in bed. *Trying to raise the arm.* At NIGHT, in bed.
< Lying on the right shoulder.
> Swinging arms to and fro. Lying on the back or on the left side.
Note: Rheumatism of parts least covered with flesh: tibia, etc.

49

SANGUINARIA CANADENSIS

▼ SYMPTOM PROFILE

Psychological
- Irritable, morose, grumbling; bad-humored in the evening.
- Anxious dread. Desire to be held. Confusion, lassitude, apathy.
- Fears that things will get worse.

Metabolic
- BURNING SENSATIONS, flushes of heat. Pulsations. Feet hot at night; sticks them out of the covers. *Burning of palms and soles.*
- *Sinking or fainting sensations with the headache.* Secretions acrid, acidic.
- Warm, wet weather causes lassitude, apathy.

Respiratory
- Lung conditions with cough, BLEEDING, shortness of breath.
- Viral bronchitis, whooping cough, *pneumonia*, croup < lying down.
- Tonsillitis, sore throats, *nasal polyps*. Asthma and HAY FEVER.

Women
- MENOPAUSAL headache, *flushes from above down*. Fibroids.

Digestive System
- Burning tongue. HEARTBURN.
- Gastritis during headache.

▼ DOSAGE

Potency
- 3 to 200. Mainly for acute phase.

Repetition
- Repeat as often as symptoms indicate.

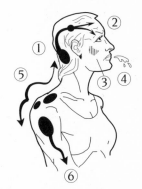

▼ CLINICAL CONDITIONS

- Bursitis (right shoulder) • Facial neuralgia • Frozen shoulder (symptomatic) • Menopausal symptoms • MIGRAINE, cluster headache, sick headache • Neck rheumatism • Neuralgia of upper jaw • Rheumatism of left hip • SHOULDER bursitis, tendonitis.

SEPIA

Ink of Cuttlefish

▼ KEYNOTES

➤ Weakness and sagging of ligaments, muscles. Depression.
➤ Low back: Tired, heavy, aching < sitting, menses, evening.
➤ Headache < lying on the back > lying on the side, heavy exertion.

▼ HEADACHE SYMPTOMS

• FOREHEAD, temples, or one side (left). Boring, bursting. Dull with inability to think. Pain like a SHOCK or blow, *jerks the head.*

• *Associated:* visual disturbances, vomiting, emptiness in stomach, DEPRESSION, anxiety, falling out of hair, chilliness, *noon till evening.*

< *Lying on back*, stooping, *motion*, cough, jar, COLD, chilling the head.

< *Menses*, menopause, *during intercourse.* Missing meals. *Artificial light.*

< A.M. on rising. After a short nap. Vomiting.

> *Lying on the painful side*, closing eyes, dark room, VIOLENT MOTION.

> OPEN AIR, after eating. REST. After a good sleep. Pressure.

(Also see modalities below under Low Back Pain)

▼ LOW BACK PAIN

• ACHING, dull pains. *Everything seems to settle in the back.*

• Burning, "as if broken," throbbing, labor-like. HEAVINESS < a.m.

• SUDDEN STITCHES, "as if struck by a hammer." Shuddering pains.

Location

• Pain in the low back, sacrum, and across the hips. Extends forward around the pelvis, to the thighs, abdomen, hips, legs. Sciatica.

• SACRAL aching, dragging pain, heaviness. Weak sacroiliac joint.

• Pain referred from uterine or pelvic conditions.

Associated

• Weak, TIRED low back < walking. Stiffness > walking.

• Spasms, jerking, twitches. Cracking joints. Frequent urination.

• Effects of overlifting, injury, blows, falls, *getting wet.*

Modalities

< SITTING, standing, stooping, leaning back, kneeling, coughing.

< Motion, rising, lifting, jarring, turning in bed, stretching, lifting.

< Morning, EVENING. Before, during, or after MENSES.

50

SEPIA OFFICINALIS

< Cold, *wet weather*, before a storm. After waking from a short nap.
> PRESSURE. *Pressing the back against, or lying upon a hard surface.*
> *Warmth*, warm bed. Drawing limbs up. Evening. Touch. Left side.
> Sitting upright. Walking in open air. Lying (on back). When busy.
• Generally > *vigorous exercise*, but NOT the low back symptoms.

▼ SYMPTOM PROFILE

Psychological

• *Depression* & weeping. Weeps when telling symptoms. Pessimistic and hopeless. Unable to show or feel affection, or to receive it.
• Intense *irritability*, easily offended. Worn down by worries and work.
• *Indifferent* to work, to pleasure, to one's loved ones. *Desires solitude.*
• Worse from sympathy, worse when alone. Better when busy.
• Dull, confused, poor memory. Lack of libido or aversion to sex.

Metabolic

• Lean, angular, narrow hips and shoulders or flabby, sagging, puffy.
• VERY CHILLY. Chronic *fatigue, weakness*. Easy or sudden FAINTING.
• Uterine and hormonal disturbances with *low back pain*, headache.

Women

• Menopause, pregnancy, dysmenorrhea, effects of the Pill, of miscarriage, during childbirth, POST-PARTUM DIFFICULTIES.
• Infertility. Uterine prolapse. *Bearing-down sensations.*

Other Systems

• Liver congestion. Prolapsed organs. Constipation.
• Empty feeling at the pit of the stomach or abdomen > eating.
• Venous problems (varicose veins, hemorrhoids).

▼ DOSAGE

Potency

• 6th to 30th in local problems. High potency in constitutional cases.

Repetition

• Need not be repeated too often.

▼ CLINICAL CONDITIONS

• Arthritis • Coccyx pain • Headache • Low back pain • Raynaud's
• Rheumatism (chronic) • Sacroiliac pain • Sciatica.

SILICEA

SiO_2

Quartz

▼ KEYNOTES

➤ HEADACHE radiating from neck and occiput to the (right) eye.
➤ NECK stiffness and pain. LOW BACK PAIN < on rising up.
➤ < Drafts, COLD air > Warmth, wrapping the head up.

▼ HEADACHE SYMPTOMS

Pain Sharp, tearing, STITCHING (both head and joints).
Location: *Occiput*. From nape of the neck to vertex, forehead and *eye*.
Associated
• Rush of blood to the head. Vertigo arising from back of head, feeling like falling forward. Weak neck. *Profuse sweat* of head, hands, feet.
Causes: Overexcitement. Mental effort or overexertion.
• COLD air or DRAFTS to the head, back, or feet.
• Headaches since a severe illness when young. *Since vaccination*.
• From suppressed foot sweat (with foot powders, etc.).

▼ MUSCULOSKELETAL SYMPTOMS

• Joints and limbs are WEAK, heavy, stiff. "Give way" easily.
• Limbs *fall asleep easily*. Destructive bone disease, fistula.
Locations
• SPINE: Spinal curvature. *Right scoliosis* with pain on motion or touch. Kyphosis. Poor posture. *Aching*, throbbing, beating, or burning pains in the mid-back, sacrum. Very sensitive to *cold or drafts*.
• NECK: Pain following low back pain. Rheumatism of the lower neck. *Weakness*. Stiffness, chilliness. Torticollis; turning is too painful.
• LOW BACK and SACRUM: Violent cramping pains < sitting, rising from a seat, stooping, jarring. Shooting down the legs or between the hips. Stiffness. *Lame feeling* in the sacrum. Chronic sciatica.
• COCCYX: Pain in the tailbone, after jarring or injury.
• LEGS: *Loss of power in the lower limbs*. Unable to rise. Hip joint disease.
• KNEES: Chronic synovitis. Swelling, ankylosis, feels as if bound.
• FEET: Cramps in the calves and soles. Severe pain in the arches.

● ●

SILICIC ACID

- HANDS: Arms heavy and weak. Fingers stiff, unable to bend.
- WRIST: Ganglia. Weakness and lameness. Contracted tendons.

Modalities

< COLD air, DRAFTS, uncovering the head. *Damp.* Weather changes.

< MOTION, stooping, RISING UP. *Jarring.* Pressure (joints).

< Night. Full or waxing moon. Menses. Noise, light.

< Mental effort, overstudy, overexertion, overwork, overstriving.

> Warmth. *Wrapping the head up warmly.* PRESSURE (headache).

▼ SYMPTOM PROFILE

Psychological

- *Lack of self-confidence.* Timid, mentally oversensitive or "porous."
- Compensates by being stubborn, with fixed opinions, conformity.
- Extremely FASTIDIOUS. Anticipation anxiety, nervousness.

Metabolic

- *Immune weakness.* Recurrent infections such as otitis, colds, etc.
- Weak, fatigued, lacks mental & physical stamina. Malassimilation.
- CHILLY. Cold hands & feet. *Restless, fidgety. Slow development,* growth.
- PERSPIRES easily, especially feet, *head,* hands. *Foul sweats.*

Skin

- Easy infection. Poor wound healing. Nails split, white spots.
- Silicea helps to reduce or absorb scar tissue.

▼ DOSAGE

Potency

- 6th to 30th in local problems. High potency for constitutional type.

Repetition

- Repeated doses of lower potencies at regular intervals.
- Single doses of higher potency for constitutional treatment.

▼ CLINICAL CONDITIONS

- Arthritic nodosities • Bone disease • Cervical pain • Coccyx pain
- Dupuytren's • Fractures (non-union) • Gout • Headache
- Knee conditions • Old injuries (to spine or coccyx) • Old sprains
- Osteophytes • Osteoporosis • Rickets • Scar tissue • Sciatica
- Scoliosis • Spina bifida • TMJ (arthritis, pain) • Torticollis
- Weak ankles.

SPIGELIA

Pinkroot

▼ KEYNOTES

➤ NEURALGIA of the head, eyes, trigeminal nerve, teeth, heart.
➤ Headache from occiput to the LEFT eye, morning till sunset.
➤ Violent, radiating pain < TOUCH, motion, jar, tobacco smoke.

▼ NEURALGIC SYMPTOMS

Pain
• Extreme, neuralgic, RADIATING pain. *Stabbing*, throbbing attacks.
• *Radiates* to all parts from within outward or below upward.

Location
• *Headache like a band*. Burrowing or bursting outward.
• OCCIPUT or neck ① to temple ② and deep into the LEFT EYE, ③ forehead, or vertex. Come and go gradually.
• Pressive pain in eyeballs; pressing outward or *drawing into brain*.
• Stiff neck and shoulders. Painful numbness < lying on the back.
• Stinging, stitching pains in the joints. Twitching of the limbs.

Associated
• HYPERSENSITIVE TO TOUCH ④. Scalp sore and sensitive.
• Eyes: red, *watery* ⑤, feel enlarged, lids heavy. Painful on motion.
• Heart palpitations. Coldness in the painful part.

Modalities
< TOUCH, MOTION. *Stooping. Jarring*. Turning the eyes. Noise.
< *Sunrise to sunset*. Noon. COLD and damp, rain. Washing. Storms.
< TOBACCO SMOKE or smoky rooms (may induce headache).
< Raising the arms. Left side. Tea.
> COLD APPLICATIONS. *After sunset*. Closing the eyes. Deep breaths.
> *Lying on the right side with the head high*.

Other Unusual Symptoms
• Bubbling sensation in the head.
• Feeling of *looseness of the brain* in the skull when turning the head.
• Swashing sensation, on shaking the head or while walking.
  (also China, Nux-v, Rhus tox, Bryonia, Belladonna, Sulphur)

52 •

SPIGELIA ANTHELMIA

▼ SYMPTOM PROFILE

Psychological
- ANXIETY with the pain or about the future. *Fear of pointed objects.*
- Fear and anxiety on deep inspiration. Anxiety felt in the chest.
- Sad and discouraged. *Stuttering and stammering.*

Metabolic
- Chilly < cold. Anemic and weak. Offensive sweats of hands / feet.
- Pale or yellow, earthy complexion. Wrinkled appearance.

Eye
- Neuralgias, pain, and aching deep in the eyes. Eyes feel too large.
- Accommodation errors. Pains of *glaucoma*. Ciliary neuralgia.

Head
- Toothache from cold air or water, or while eating.
- Vertigo on looking down, turning the eyes, stooping > lying.

Cardiovascular
- Pericarditis, palpitations. ANGINA. Hyperthyroid tachycardia.
- Violent sticking pains radiating to the arm, back, or throat.

▼ DOSAGE

Potency
- 6th to 30th.

Repetition
- Long-lasting effects.
- Very infrequent repetition needed.

▼ CLINICAL CONDITIONS

- *Chronic pain syndromes* • Exopthalmic goiter • Jaw pain • Migraine
- Neuralgia: *Trigeminal or facial neuralgia* (main remedy), dental neuralgia, ciliary neuralgia, herpetic neuralgia (shingles) of the face
- Parasites or roundworms (in children) • Rheumatic disease of the eye or heart • Stitches in the diaphragm • *Tension headache* • Vertigo.

STAPHYSAGRIA

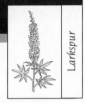

Larkspur

▼ KEYNOTES

➤ Effects of suppressed anger, indignation, humiliation.
➤ Cutting wounds or lacerations, especially to abdomen, genitals.
➤ Low back pain in the morning, as if broken > motion.

▼ MUSCULOSKELETAL SYMPTOMS

Pain

• SORE, bruised, beaten, as if sprained. Stinging. Shifting pains.
• Stitching, tearing, and drawing pains and sensations.
• Tender and sensitive: Muscles pain < touch. Joints < motion.

Modalities

< TOUCH, stretching. Motion (except back, that is > motion).
< Insults, humiliation or indignation, frustration. Suppressed anger.
> Warmth, rest, night. Hard pressure. Lying or sitting.

Associated

• Limbs feel bruised and *very weak*.
• STIFF JOINTS in the morning on rising.
• Skin symptoms may alternate with joint pain.
• Cough may alternate with sciatica.

Locations

• LOW BACK: Pain *in bed in the morning, as if sprained* or broken.
  < Rest, touch, rising from a seat, sitting, turning, night.
  > Standing, walking. Stitches radiating upward.
• NECK: Tension, pressure, or drawing pains in the neck with *stiffness*.
• SHOULDER: Pain as if sprained < motion, touch.
• HANDS: *Arthritic nodes*. Inflammation and pain of the fingertips.
  Knuckle joints, finger joints, and tips affected < left index finger.
• LEGS: *Crural neuralgia*. Aching of buttocks extending to the hip joint
  and small of the back. Restless legs with pains in the calves.
• KNEES: Weak knees. *Stitches*, burning pains in the hollow of the
  knees. Contraction of muscles in the back of the knees.

53

DELPHINIUM STAPHYSAGRIA

Trauma
- Wounds by sharp instruments (knife, glass). Cuts and lacerations.
- Post-surgical pain, after a major abdominal operation.
- Stretched or wounded body orifices (rectum, vagina). *Stitching pain.*
- CORNEA INJURY. Neuralgia after tooth extraction.

▼ SYMPTOM PROFILE

Psychological
- Effects of humiliation, insults. *Indignation.* SUPPRESSED ANGER.
- ANGER: throws things, rage, suspiciousness. Self-righteous anger.
- Unable to express emotions: shy, mild, sweet, or restrained.

Head
- HEAVY sensation in forehead. Head as if squeezed. Tearing pain.
- < Motion > Rest, warmth, YAWNING.

Skin
- Formication; crawling and itching, *changes place on scratching.*
- Eczema, psoriasis. Fleshy warts.

Genitourinary
- Cystitis, from intercourse or during pregnancy. Salpingitis.
- Effects of excess masturbation or sexual activity. Prostatitis.

Face
- TOOTHACHE, tooth decay, causing neuralgia in the face and head.
- Styes, chalazion. Abrasions to the cornea.

▼ DOSAGE

Potency
- 3rd to 30th. Higher if the emotional symptoms correspond well.

Repetition
- Repeat as required by symptoms.

▼ CLINICAL CONDITIONS

> - Acute rheumatism • Arthritic nodosities • Chronic GOUT with nodosities in the hands and feet with much swelling
> - Hip joint disease • Knee pain • Osteitis (bone inflammation)
> - Sciatica (< motion) • .Scoliosis • Thoracic kyphosis
> - Wounds (cuts, lacerations).

STELLARIA

Chickweed

▼ **KEYNOTES**

➤ ARTHRITIS, acute or chronic (similar to Pulsatilla).
➤ Joint pain and inflammation, WANDERING from joint to joint.
➤ Stitching pains. < Heat, touch > Motion, cool air, cool bathing.

▼ **MUSCULOSKELETAL SYMPTOMS**

Pain

• STITCHING, sharp, darting. Erratic, shifting, wandering pains.
• WANDERING inflammation or pain, moving from the hip to the thighs, ankle, foot, arm, wrist, etc.
• SORENESS to touch. Bruised sensation.
• Pains appear suddenly, gradually or slowly reach a maximum, and finally stop suddenly.

Associated

• NODOSITIES. Finger joints enlarged. Gouty deposits of hands, feet.
• SYNOVITIS: Subacute or chronic rheumatism or *joint inflammation*.
• Stiffness. Numbness. Swelling.

Specific Locations

• Arthritis or synovitis of the knee, ankle, shoulder, hip, finger joints.
• NECK: Pain and stiffness with pain down the arms into the index finger (of the left hand). Pain under the right shoulder blade.
• LOW BACK: Lancinating pains. Sharp pains over the buttocks, radiating to the thighs and legs < stooping.
Aching pain in the kidney region with weariness, lameness.
Bruised feeling in the thighs from exertion.
• HEAD: Dull frontal headache with drowsiness < morning.

Modalities

< HEAT, warmth of the bed.
< Morning. TOUCH. Rest. Tobacco use.
> MOTION, walking. Open air, cool air. Sea air.
> Cold or tepid bathing. Bathing in sea water, lake, or river water.
> Evening (6-9 p.m.)

54 •

STELLARIA MEDIA

▼ SYMPTOM PROFILE

Psychological
- IRRITABLE.
- Fatigue, lethargy. No desire to work.

Metabolic
- General congestion. SLUGGISH, sleepiness in the morning.
- Chilly. Emaciation. Venous stasis or congestion.

Abdomen
- Liver congestion or enlargement with sensitivity to touch.
- Lancinating, stitching pains. Clay-colored feces. Nausea.
- Constipation or alternating constipation and diarrhea.
- Whole abdomen is sore and tender to touch.

Other Symptoms
- Protruding eyes.
- Numbness of the tip of the tongue.
- Psoriasis.

▼ DOSAGE

Potency
- Low potencies (2x traditionally, but up to the 30th may be used).
- The tincture may be used simultaneously on affected joints.

Repetition
- Repeat low potencies three times daily for up to one month.

▼ CLINICAL CONDITIONS

- Arthritis • Gout • Headache • Low back pain • Neck pain with radiculitis • Nodosities • Polyarthritis • Rheumatism • Synovitis.

STICTA

Lungwort

▼ KEYNOTES

➤ Synovitis, bursitis, rheumatism of the knee, shoulder, neck, wrist.
➤ Swelling, heat, redness in spots. Cold sweat of hands, feet.
➤ < Motion, night, touch, right side > Daytime.

▼ MUSCULOSKELETAL SYMPTOMS

Pain

• Darting pains in various joints of the limbs. Intense pains prevent sleep. Sharp, lancinating pains in the knee, fingers, elbows, etc.
• Pains spreading from area to area until every joint is involved.
• *Causes*: After-effects of a fall. After chilling or respiratory problems.

Locations

• SYNOVITIS, BURSITIS, acute or subacute rheumatism or arthritis of the *neck, shoulder, wrists, knee, ankles*. Large and small joints.
• NECK: *Stiffness* and pain of the vertebrae and muscles radiating to the shoulder, arms, fingers. Soreness. Unable to put one's coat on.
• SHOULDER: Right shoulder bursitis with pain in the deltoid, extending into the biceps and arms.
• WRISTS: Swollen, painful on motion.
• KNEE: Inflammation with shooting pains.
  Swelling, edema and redness, sore to the touch.
• ANKLE: Rheumatism with swelling and intense pain.

Associated

• SWELLING, heat, redness of joints. Severe drawing pains.
• Circumscribed *red or inflamed spots over the joint*.
• Legs feel *as if floating in the air*. Restless limbs, hands, feet.
• Profuse sweating of hands and / or feet. Cold and clammy.

Modalities

< MOTION (though the knee may be better from stretching).
< NIGHT. Lying down. Changes of temperature. *Right side*. TOUCH.
> Daytime. Rheumatism is > as the day advances.
> Open air. After a discharge commences.

55
• •

STICTA PULMONARIA

▼ SYMPTOM PROFILE

Psychological
- Nervous, LOQUACIOUS — feels compelled to talk about anything.
- Dullness, lassitude, lethargy.
- Peculiar sensation of levitation, of floating in the air.

Metabolic
- Burning or sticking pains all over the body.

Nose and throat
- Allergy. Rhinitis. Sinusitis. Hay fever. Influenza.
- Nasal membranes and air passages *extremely dry*.
- Crusts and mucus plugs in the nose.
- Nasal obstruction. Urging to blow the nose, but no discharge.
- Headache with fullness and heavy pressure at the root of the nose.
- Constant sneezing. Post-nasal drip. Tingling of the nose.

Respiratory
- Dry hacking cough with *tickling* in the throat and larynx. N*ight cough*.
- Worse from inspiration or when tired. Croup.

Sleep
- Insomnia from nervousness or cough. After surgery. *After fractures*.

▼ DOSAGE

Potency
- Generally low potencies: 6th or 12th.

Repetition
- Hourly in acute phase; otherwise two to three times daily.

▼ CLINICAL CONDITIONS

> - Ankle rheumatism • Arthritis • Bursitis • Knee bursitis (House-
> maid's knee) • Restless leg syndrome • Shoulder rheumatism
> - Synovitis • Torticollis • Wrist rheumatism.

STRONTIUM CARB

$SrCO_3$

Strontium Carbonate

▼ KEYNOTES

➤ Weak and SWOLLEN ankles. Chronic sprain of ankles (or wrist).
➤ Gnawing, TEARING pain. Sudden deep bone pain.
➤ < COLD, walking, evening & night, rubbing > HEAT in any form.

▼ MUSCULOSKELETAL SYMPTOMS

Pain

• Fleeting pains. TEARING, burning, gnawing, stitching, drawing.
• Deep pain in the *marrow of bones*. Increase and decrease gradually.

Location

• ANKLE pain and weakness. Chronic or recurrent joint sprains.
• Rheumatism or old injuries of WRISTS, *hips, knees*, or *shoulder* with pain symptoms and modalities of Strontium carb.
• To a lesser degree, may be indicated for elbows, fingers, or feet.
• Neck pain > wrapping up warmly. *Chills the in back, in the lumbar spine.*
• *Low back pain*: Sore, gnawing, drawing < sitting, walking, at stool.

Associated

• SWOLLEN ANKLES and feet. Swelling long after a sprain.
• *Icy cold feet*. Feet burning at night. Muscles twitching in sleep.
• *Paralytic weakness* of the limbs, of one side (right). Twitching, jerking.
• Pains and weakness of the legs at night in bed > motion of legs.
• Hands numb, sore, with crawling sensations.
• *Cramping* in calves, soles. Coldness in spots on calves.
• Feel ill all over with the pain. Pain alternates with itching.
• Diarrhea with the rheumatism.

Modalities

< COLD, uncovering, undressing. DRAFTS. Weather changes.
< WALKING, exertion. *Sitting*. Stooping. Standing. *Rising from lying*.
< *Rubbing*. Touch. RIGHT SIDE. *Evening*, NIGHT, in bed.
> HEAT: *warm bath*, wrapping up warmly, warm bed, *radiant heat*.
> Light. Sun (heat and light). Open air.

STRONTIUM CARBONICUM

▼ SYMPTOM PROFILE

Psychological

- FEAR and anxiety. Easily startled < at night in bed, a.m.
- ANGER: Silent, taciturn with violent outbursts of temper and striking out at others. Irritable, quarrelsome, malicious.
- Insomnia. Startled on falling to sleep. Nightmares with crying out.
- *Depression, gloom*; a.m. on waking and evening in bed. Poor memory.

Metabolic

- CHILLY. Aversion to darkness > light. Night sweats.
- Shock after surgical operations. Effects of hemorrhage.
- Great emaciation.

Head

- Congestion to head with *heat of the head and face*. Face flushed, bright red, yet averse to uncovering and > wrapping warmly.
- Headache from tension in the neck, extending forward to the head.

Circulatory

- Arteriosclerosis, high blood pressure. Menopausal flushing.
- *Tendency to stroke*. Hemiplegia.

▼ DOSAGE

Potency

- Low potencies, up to the 30th, though some recommend 200c.

Repetition

- Infrequent repetitions.

▼ CLINICAL CONDITIONS

- Ankle sprain • Ankle weakness • Bone disease or osteitis (femur)
- Eye surgery • Flat feet • Gout • Growing pains • Headache
- Hip joint disease • Neuritis < cold • Rheumatism of larger joints
- Sciatica (with swelling of the ankle) • Shoulder rheumatism
- Sprains (chronic or recurrent) • TRAUMA (long term effects of dislocations, sprains, severe injury) • Wrist arthritis.

SULPHUR

S

Brimstone

▼ KEYNOTES

➤ Back pain < bending, MOTION, rising up. Unable to stand erect.
➤ Neck pain with stiffness, cracking on extension < motion, night.
➤ Joints inflamed, weak, and stiff. BURNING, tearing pains.

▼ MUSCULOSKELETAL SYMPTOMS

- PAINS: Various: drawing, stitching, burning, tearing, or bruised.
- INFLAMED JOINTS, with much redness, swelling, intense pain on motion, *travels from above downward*. Cramping and contracture.
- WEAKNESS of joints and muscles. Trembling. Uneasy feeling.
- STIFF JOINTS with deposits. CRACKING joints. *Follows Bryonia well.*

Spine

- Sensation of the vertebrae sliding over one another.
- Spinal curvature. Coldness and chills in the spine. Cracking.
- *Stoop-shouldered posture*. Sits slumped, walks slouched.
- Supports weight on his hands when sitting.
- NECK: Stiffness. Cracking joints on bending backward. Drawing, tearing, stitching pains. Torticollis. Pain radiates into the shoulder.
- THORAX: Drawing, aching, *tension* between the scapulae < lying.
- LOW BACK: Burning, stitching, or bruised pain. Stiffness. Cracking. *Pain on rising. Unable to stand erect* or straighten. < Stooping, moving.
- Sacrum and coccyx pain. Back feels shortened or contracted.

Extremities

- SHOULDER rheumatism (left). Lacerating pains < night, lying on it, rest, on first motion > continued motion.
- ELBOW: *Tearing pain* > motion. Pain from 11 p.m. to 7 a.m. Tension.
- Tearing pain in arms and hands. Trembling or numbness of hands.
- WRIST: As if sprained. Stiff, swollen < slight motion > fast motion.
- HIP: Violent pain < motion, touch, walking. Sudden cramps. Drawing, bruised pains in thighs. *Shooting pain* < rest > motion, pressure.
- KNEE: Pain, swelling, stiffness, cracking. Tightness in hollow of the knees. Cramps in the calves at night. Rheumatism of *ankles and feet*.

57

SULPHUR SUBLIMATUM

Modalities

< STANDING ERECT, straightening. *Stooping*. Rising up. After sitting.

< Motion, jarring, lifting, coughing, WALKING, turning.

(Back and many limb pains are < motion, some are relieved.)

< WARM room or bed. After suppression of skin eruptions.

< NIGHT, evening, or midday. Every 24 hours, or once every week.

< *Touch*. Weather changes. Wet weather. Cold bathing, getting wet.

> Motion (sciatica, tearing in wrist, elbow, legs, shooting in hips).

> Dry weather. Lying on the right side.

▼ **SYMPTOM PROFILE**

Psychological

• *Intellectual* and philosophical or materialistic and earthy in outlook.

• LAZINESS. Sloppy or unkempt. Dislikes standing, sits slouched.

• Self-confident or arrogant. Critical, fault-finding. Argumentative.

• Selfish and cynical or extroverted, generous. Anxiety about health.

Note: There is a wide variety of "Sulphur types"— it is used for the broadest possible range of physical and mental conditions.

Metabolic

• Lack of REACTION to remedies. Poor vitality or immune response.

• Great tiredness and lethargy. Hunger at 11 a.m. Foul perspiration.

• Warm-blooded. Hands and feet chilly, yet burning and heat of feet or hands. Sticks them out of the covers at night. Averse to bathing.

Skin: Eruptions with intense itching and burning < scratching.

▼ **DOSAGE**

Potency

• 12 or 30 in local conditions. High potency for constitutional type.

Repetition

• Daily doses for acute or local disease. Single dose of high potency.

▼ **CLINICAL CONDITIONS**

• Arthritis • Brachial neuralgia • Bursitis • Coccyx pain • Gout • Hip joint disease • Knee synovitis • Kyphosis • Low back pain • Neck pain • Rheumatoid arthritis • Sciatica • Scoliosis • Shoulder rheumatism • Torticollis • Wrist ganglion.

SYMPHYTUM

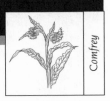

Comfrey

▼ KEYNOTES

➤ Trauma to bone and periosteum or to the eye. Bone disease.
➤ Fracture: accelerates bone healing time. Bone inflammation.
➤ Prickling pain at the site of old wounds, fractures, or amputation.

▼ MUSCULOSKELETAL CONDITIONS

Pain
• PRICKLING, stitching. Little bruising generally.

Location
• PERIOSTEUM. BONES. Cartilage, tendon, joints.
• Pain in area of bony protuberances: elbow, epicondyles, ankles.

Modalities
< Touch, motion, pressure.
> Gentle motion, warmth.

Trauma
• Pain at the site of OLD WOUNDS or FRACTURES, past injury to cartilage or bone.
• Injuries from blunt instruments.
• Post-surgical pain at the site of amputation or bone puncture.
• Arnica for soft tissue injury, Symphytum for injury to hard tissue.

Bone
• FRACTURE. Comminuted fracture. NON-UNION OF BONES.
• Accelerates the formation of callus. *Reduces healing time by half.*
• *Bone inflammation*, periostitis with pain and soreness.
• Osteoporosis. Brittle bones.
• Injury to periosteum.
• Symphytum has a reputation for the treatment of bone cancers.

Musculoskeletal
• Skull fracture or head injury (compare Hypericum, Nat sulph).
• Spinal injury.
• Psoas abscess.
• Low back pain from injury, overexertion, or excess sexual activity.
• Knee arthralgia • Tennis elbow.

• •

SYMPHYTUM OFFICINALE

▼ SYMPTOM PROFILE

Eye
- Injuries or blows to the *eyeball* (main remedy), eye socket, or sclera.
- Retinal bleeding. Bleeding inside the eye after injury.
- Traumatic conjunctivitis.
- Long-lasting pain or soreness in the eye after injury.

Teeth
- Periodontal disease.

Face
- Cancer of the antrum of the face.
- Facial injury.

Digestive
- Gastric ulcer (low potency).

▼ DOSAGE

Potency
- Lower potencies (3-12), though 30c once a day has been used very successfully. Occasional doses of 200c can also be used.
- Tincture (ø) can be used externally in any musculoskeletal condition listed above or for sores, ulcers, swellings.

Repetition
- Frequent repetition; can be used for weeks or months.

▼ CLINICAL CONDITIONS

- Bone injury • Eye injury • Fracture • Gingivitis • Low back pain
- Osteoporosis • Pain at site of old wounds or fractures • Periostitis
- Tennis elbow • Trauma to bone, amputation.

TELLURIUM

Te

Tellurium

▼ KEYNOTES

➤ RIGHT-sided SCIATICA < cough, sneeze, jar, straining at stool.
➤ Low back or sacral pains radiating into right leg. Disc syndrome.
➤ Sensitive to TOUCH; sensitive in bones, in thoracic spine.

▼ MUSCULOSKELETAL SYMPTOMS

Pain
- Sudden, radiating pains. Burning pains. Come and go suddenly.
- Sharp, quick pains, followed by soreness.

Location
- *Low back pain* or sacral pain extending to the RIGHT thigh and leg.
- Sciatica, but particularly RIGHT-SIDED SCIATICA.
- *Thorax*: Upper thoracic spine sensitive (C7-T5), with pain radiating to the head, neck, shoulder, or sternum < fatigue > rest.
- *Leg*: Hip and knee sore, bruised, as if sprained. Ankle rheumatism.
- *Upper limbs*: Rheumatism of the elbow, hands.
  Finger numbness on stretching out the hands.
- One-sided symptoms (especially the right side).

Associated
- Spine and joints SENSITIVE TO TOUCH, causing radiating pain.
- Soreness and tenderness.
- Numbness of the neck, occiput.
- Contraction of tendons and muscles of the leg, bends of the knees.
- Effects of injury to the spine or sacrum.
- Limbs heavy, tired.

Modalities
< COUGHING, *jarring*, *laughing*, *sneezing*, STRAINING at stool.
< TOUCH, pressure, friction. Cold.
< NIGHT. Weekly.
< Stooping, lying or *lying on the painful area*, right side.
> Walking, lying on the back, flexing the leg. Open air. Urination.

TELLURIUM

▼ **SYMPTOM PROFILE**

Psychological
- Cheerful and gay, followed by impatience, irritability.
- Hypersensitive and excitable with violent anger, temper tantrums.
- Dull, absent-minded and forgetful, especially about business.
- Fears approach of others, of BEING TOUCHED in sensitive places.

Metabolic
- Weakness and lassitude. Drowsiness.
- All discharges acrid, offensive, with *fish-brine odor.*
- Foul perspiration. *Offensive foot perspiration.*

Head
- Left-sided headache, above the forehead and the left eye.

Eyes, Ears
- Eyes puffy, eczema of the lids. Conjunctivitis, cataract.
- OTITIS with fetid or acrid discharge. Eczema behind the ears.

Skin
- RINGWORM of the whole body, or around the anus or perineum, breasts, hair follicles. Circular eruptions. Itching when warm < night.
- Psoriasis.

▼ **DOSAGE**

Potency
- 6th to 30th.

Repetition
- Long-acting; needs infrequent repetition.

▼ **CLINICAL CONDITIONS**

- Acute disc syndrome
- Head injury.
- Lumbar neuralgia
- SCIATICA (right-sided).
- Thoracic neuralgia, myalgia, subluxation
- Trauma: to the spine or sacrum.

THIOSINAMINUM

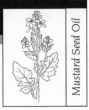

Mustard Seed Oil

▼ **KEYNOTES**

➤ DISSOLVING OF SCAR TISSUE in any area of the body.
➤ Stiffness, restriction, contracture of joints, tendons, ligaments.
➤ Residual effects of injuries, inflammation, burns. Tinnitus.

▼ **CLINICAL CONDITIONS**

Musculoskeletal
• Scar tissue, ADHESIONS, cicatrices. Keloids.
• Adhesions of JOINTS, after *inflammation or injury* in arthritis.
• Adhesions in LIGAMENT and tendon. Ankylosis.
• STIFFNESS of joints.
• Frozen shoulder.
• Painful adhesions (stretch pain) in any joint.
• Tennis elbow (adhesions in the brachialis muscle, etc.).
• Carpal tunnel syndrome (thickening of the restraining ligaments).
• Dupuytren's contracture.

Metabolic
• Senile dementia or premature aging. To retard old age.
• Contracture of skin, tendons, ligaments after burns.
• Arteriosclerosis.
• Tumors or enlarged glands. Fibroid tumors.

Eye
• Cataract of the lens or cornea.
• Stricture of the lachrymal duct.

Ear
• Adhesions of the eustachian tube.
• Thickening of the ear drum. Otosclerosis.
• Otitis media. Eustachian tube catarrh.
• MENIERE'S SYNDROME, vertigo.
• TINNITUS AURIUM.

ALLYL SULPHOCARBAMIDE

Abdomen
- Internal adhesions after surgery, after hysterectomy, etc.
- Intestinal strictures. Stricture of the rectum.
- Pyloric stenosis.
- Stricture of the urethra.

Skin
- Scleroderma. Lupus.
- Keloids (excess scarring after injury).
- Scarring from cosmetic surgery, breast implants, etc.

Genitourinary
- Uterine fibroma.
- Prostatic enlargement.

Nervous system
- Locomotor ataxia. Alzheimer's disease.

DOSAGE

Potency
- 1x, 2x, 3x, 6x are most commonly used. Can be used externally simultaneously. If several tablets or pellets are dissolved in spring water, some can be applied topically, and the rest taken orally.

Repetition
- Three times daily for several weeks or months. Useful to alternate with other scar tissue remedies in low potency, such as Silicea, Calcarea fluor, Graphites, or Causticum, according to indications.

Note: An *important remedy for gradual reduction or dissolution of scar tissue or adhesions internally and externally, and on both gross and microscopic levels. Though few psychological symptoms, metabolic symptoms, or modalities are known as yet, Thiosinaminum's action in the above conditions is well verified.*

VIOLA

Sweet Violet

▼ **KEYNOTES**

➤ Right WRIST, ankle, or shoulder inflammation. Carpal tunnel.
➤ Pressing, BURNING pains. TENSION, heat. TREMBLING parts.
➤ < MOTION, cold air, before rising > After rising.

▼ **MUSCULOSKELETAL SYMPTOMS**

Pain and Locations

• WRIST: Rheumatism of the right wrist, carpal tunnel syndrome. Pressing pain in the right hand and finger joints.
Radiation of pain up towards the arm, or pain felt simultaneously in the right shoulder tip. Drawing pain in the elbows.
Swelling of wrist, hands, and fingers with burning pains and HEAT. Hand held immobile, half-flexed on the forearm.
Perspiration of the palm, stiffness of the hand.
• SHOULDER: Rheumatism, felt in the right deltoid area.
• KNEE: Right ankle or knee painful, swollen < least motion.
• NECK: *Tension* and drawing pain near the nape of the neck, extending downward in the evening. Weak neck.
• HEAD: Tension of the scalp, from neck and occiput to forehead and upper face < bending forward or backward. *Wrinkles forehead or knits brows with the pain.* Pain above the eyebrows. Burning in forehead.

Associated

• TREMBLING of the affected part or of whole upper limb.
• BURNING SENSATIONS, flying, changing place, like a flame.
• Stretching and yawning. KNITS THE BROWS TOGETHER.
• *Tension felt everywhere.* Numbness, weakness, debility.
• Bruised pain in bed in the morning after rising.

Modalities

< MOTION. Sitting, WALKING.
< COLD AIR, cold room. Cloudy weather, damp. Dry cold. Open air.
< In the morning, BEFORE RISING. Right side.

● ●

VIOLA ODORATA

< Lying, lying in bed. Lying on, or pressure on the *painless* side.
> AFTER RISING in the morning. Warm weather.
> Massage, energy work, hypnosis ("magnetism").

▼ SYMPTOM PROFILE

Psychological
• Mind very clear, with abundant ideas and thoughts. Intellectual.
• Confusion, with fragmented and vanishing thoughts; forgets the beginning of the sentence, etc. Unstable, unsettled state.
• Hysterical. Weeping without cause. Childish behavior.

Metabolic
• More often indicated in women, dark-haired people.
• Bedwetting or worms in children.

Eyes, Ears.
• Conditions with ear, eye, and kidney symptoms together.
• Otitis with discharge. Choroiditis. AVERSION TO MUSIC.

Sleep
• Yawning and stretching without sleepiness. Insomnia.
• Sleeps with the knees drawn up. With hands over the head.

Chest
• Constriction. Stitching pain. Dyspnea with anxiety, palpitations.

▼ DOSAGE

Potency
• From the first to the 30th potency.

Repetition
• Repeat daily or as required by symptoms.

▼ CLINICAL CONDITIONS

• Ankle rheumatism • Carpal tunnel syndrome • Ciliary neuralgia
• Headache (forehead) • Shoulder rheumatism • TMJ problems
• WRIST inflammation or arthritis.

Therapeutic Guide

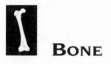

BONE

Bone Pain

Agaricus, Argentum nit, Arnica, Arsenicum, Belladonna, Berberis, Calc carb, Calc phos, Chamomilla, Cocculus, COLCHICUM, Colocynthis, Fluoric acid, Gelsemium, Kalmia, Lycopodium, MERCURIUS, Nat sulph, Phosphorus, Phytolacca, PULSATILLA, Rhododendron, RUTA, Sepia, Silicea, Staphysagria, STRONTIUM CARB, Sulphur, Symphytum, Tellurium.

Bone Spurs / Osteophytes / Nodosities

Calc carb, CALC FLUOR, Calc phos, Caulophyllum, Causticum, Colchicum, Dulcamara, Formica rufa, Guaiacum, HECLA LAVA, Phytolacca, Rhododendron, Rhus tox (for symptoms only; will not remove spurs), Ruta, Silicea, Stellaria.

Growing Pains

Agaricus, Calc carb, CALC PHOS, Causticum, Cimicifuga, Colchicum, GUAIACUM, Phosphoric acid, Phosphorus, Silicea, STRONTIUM CARB.

Osteitis

Belladonna, Bryonia, Calc carb, Calc phos, Formica rufa, HECLA LAVA, Lycopodium, MERCURIUS, Phytolacca, Pulsatilla, Ruta, SILICEA, Staphysagria, Strontium carb, Sulphur, Symphytum.

Osteomalacia (Rickets)

CALC CARB, Calc fluor, CALC PHOS, Formica rufa, Guaiacum, Hecla lava, SILICEA, Symphytum.

Osteoporosis

CALC CARB, Calc fluor, CALC PHOS, Phosphorus, Silicea, Strontium carb, Symphytum.

Periostitis

Fluoric acid, Formica rufa, Guaiacum, Hecla lava, MERCURIUS, Phosphoric acid, Phytolacca, RUTA, SILICEA, Staphysagria, SYMPHYTUM.

Tumors

AURUM, CALC FLUOR, Calc phos, Colocynthis, Dulcamara, Formica rufa, HECLA LAVA, Phytolacca, Pulsatilla, Rhododendron, Rhus tox, Ruta, SILICEA, Sulphur, Thiosinaminum.

CONNECTIVE TISSUE

Connective Tissue Disease
APIS, Argentum nit, *Bryonia*, CALC CARB, Colchicum, Dulcamara, Kali carb, Lycopodium, Nat sulph, Pulsatilla, RHUS TOX, Sepia, *Silicea*, SULPHUR.

Dupuytren's Contracture
CALC FLUOR, CAUSTICUM, Formic acid, Gelsemium, Graphites, GUAIACUM, Nat mur, SILICEA, THIOSINAMINUM.

Ligaments
BRYONIA, CALC FLUOR, *Causticum*, *Chamomilla*, *Cimicifuga*, Colchicum, Guaiacum, Kali carb, Lycopodium, Phytolacca, Pulsatilla, Rhododendron, RHUS TOX, Sepia (weak ligaments), Silicea.

Scar Tissue
CALC FLUOR, Calendula (prevention), *Causticum*, GRAPHITES, Hypericum (pain), *Phytolacca*, Ranunculus (pain from adhesions), SILICEA, THIOSINAMINUM.

Scarring after Injury (Excessive Scarring)
ARSENICUM, Bellis, *Calc carb*, *Calendula*, Carbo veg, Causticum, FLUORIC ACID, GRAPHITES, Hepar sulph, Hypericum, *Lachesis*, Nux vomica, Phosphorus, Phytolacca, Rhus tox, SILICEA, Sulphuric acid, Sulphur, Thiosinaminum, Thuja.

Sclerosis, Fibrosis
Calc fluor, Causticum, Hecla lava, Phytolacca, Silicea.

Tendonitis (Inflammation of tendons)
Bryonia, Calc phos, Causticum, Chelidonium, *Cimicifuga*, *Guaiacum*, Hypericum, Ledum, PHYTOLACCA, Pulsatilla, *Rhododendron*, RHUS TOX, Ruta, Sanguinaria.

Tendons
Ammonium mur, Calc carb, Calc fluor, CAUSTICUM, Guaiacum, Ledum, Lycopodium, Nat sulph, Nux vomica, Phytolacca, Rhododendron, RHUS TOX, RUTA, Silicea, Tellurium, Thiosinaminum.

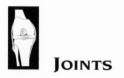

JOINTS

Ankylosis (Fusion of bone)
Calc fluor, Calc phos, *Causticum*, Colchicum, Rhus tox, *Silicea*, Sulphur, Thiosinaminum.

Arthritic Nodosities
(see Nodosities under Bone)

Arthritis
(see Osteoarthritis, Rheumatoid arthritis)

Bursitis
Acute: APIS, Belladonna, Bryonia, Pulsatilla, RHUS TOX, RUTA.
Chronic: Calc fluor, Calc phos, Nat mur, Phytolacca, Rhododendron, Sanguinaria, SILICEA., Strontium carb, Sulphur.

Contraction of Joints, Tendons, Muscles
Ammonium mur, Bellis, Calc carb, Calc phos, CAUSTICUM, Cimicifuga, Colocynthis, Formica rufa, Gelsemium, GUAIACUM, NAT MUR, Nux vomica, Phytolacca, Rhus tox, Ruta, Sepia, Staphysagria, Sulphur, Tellurium, Thiosinaminum.

Cracking / Crepitus
Aconitum, Agaricus, Ammonium carb, *Benzoic acid*, *Calc carb*, Calc fluor, Caulophyllum, *Causticum*, *Chamomilla*, *Cocculus*, *Ferrum*, *Kali bich*, *Kali carb*, Kalmia, Lachnantes, LEDUM, *Lycopodium*, *Nat mur*, *Nat sulph*, *Nux vomica*, *Phosphorus*, RHUS TOX, Ruta, *Sepia*, *Sulphur*, *Thuja*.

Gout
Berberis, CHINA, Colchicum, *Guaiacum*, Kalmia, Ledum, LYCOPODIUM, Phytolacca, Pulsatilla, Rhododendron, Spigelia, Sulphur

Joint Inflammation:
ACONITUM, APIS, Arnica, BELLADONNA, BRYONIA, *Calcarea*, Caulophyllum, *Causticum*, Dulcamara, *Guaiacum*, Hypericum, *Kali carb*, *Kalmia*, Lachesis, LEDUM, *Lycopodium*, *Nat mur*, *Nat sulph*, *Phytolacca*, *Pulsatilla*, *Rhododendron*, *Rhus tox*, Ruta, *Sepia*, SILICEA, *Sulphur*.

Osteoarthritis

Calc carb, Calc phos, Causticum, Formica rufa, Guaiacum, Ledum, *Phytolacca*, Rhododendron, Rhus tox, Ruta (see specific areas).

Polyarthritis

Pulsatilla, Stellaria.

Rheumatoid Arthritis

Aconitum, Belladonna, Bryonia, *Phytolacca*, Pulsatilla, Rhus tox, Stellaria.

Sprains & Strains

Acute: Bryonia, Rhus tox, RUTA.

Chronic: Calc carb.

Recurrent: Calc fluor, Ledum.

Subluxation

Acute: Arnica, Bryonia, Hypericum, Rhus tox.

Chronic/Recurrent: Calc carb, Cimicifuga, RHUS TOX, Ruta.

(see sections under spine, cervical and low back, etc.)

Synovitis

Aconitum, Apis, *Arnica*, Belladonna, Berberis, Bryonia, Calc carb, Calc fluor, Causticum, Fluoric acid, Kali carb, Ledum, Lycopodium, Nat mur, Phytolacca, *Pulsatilla*, Rhus tox, Ruta, Sepia, *Silicea*, STELLARIA, *Sticta*, Sulphur.

Tendonitis, Tenosynovitis

Bryonia, Causticum, Guaiacum, *Phytolacca*, Rhododendron, Rhus tox.

Weak Joints (Ligamentous laxity)

Aconitum, Actea spicata, Bryonia, Calc carb, Calc fluor, Causticum, Kali carb, Ledum, Lycopodium, Nat mur, Pulsatilla, RHUS TOX, Ruta, SEPIA, *Silicea*, Sulphur, Thuja.

MUSCLE

Fibromyalgia, Fibrositis
Bryonia, Calc carb, *Causticum*, CIMICIFUGA, Formica rufa, *Guaiacum*, Kali bich, *Kalmia*, Nux vomica, Phosphorus, PHYTOLACCA, Ranunculus, RHUS TOX, RUTA, Silicea.

Muscle Strains / Injuries
ARNICA, BELLIS, Calc carb, Nat carb, Nat mur, Phosphorus, RHUS TOX.

Myalgia, Myositis (Muscle pain and inflammation)
Aconitum, ARNICA, *Belladonna*, BRYONIA, Causticum, CIMICIFUGA, *Dulcamara*, *Gelsemium*, Hecla lava, *Phytolacca*, Ranunculus, Rhododendron, RHUS TOX, Sanguinaria, Tellurium.

Spasm, Cramps
Actea spicata, *Agaricus*, Arsenicum, Belladonna, Calc carb, Calc fluor, Calc phos, Causticum, CHAMOMILLA, CIMICIFUGA, Cocculus, COLOCYNTHIS, Cuprum, Formica rufa, Gelsemium (writer's cramp), Gnaphalium, Iris vers, Kalmia, Ledum, Lycopodium, Nat mur, NUX VOMICA, Phytolacca, Ranunculus, Rhus tox, Silicea, Strontium carb, Sulphur.

Tenderness
Apis, BRYONIA, CIMICIFUGA, Colchicum, Phytolacca, Ruta.

Tension, muscular
ACONITUM, Ammonium mur, Arnica, Arsenicum, Belladonna, Berberis, Causticum, Dulcamara, *Guaiacum*, Kali carb, Lachesis, Ledum, *Nat carb*, *Nat mur*, NITRIC ACID, NUX VOMICA, PHOSPHORUS, Phytolacca, *Pulsatilla*, *Rhus tox*, SEPIA, *Silicea*, Staphysagria, Sulphur.

Weakness of Muscles
Aconitum, Agaricus, Arsenicum, Belladonna, Berberis, Bryonia, *Calc carb*, Causticum, Chamomilla, Cimicifuga, Cocculus, Colchicum, *Dulcamara*, Ferrum, GELSEMIUM, Kali carb, Lycopodium, NAT MUR, Nux vomica, Phosphorus, *Plumbum*, Pulsatilla, Ranunculus, *Rhododendron*, *Sepia*, *Silicea*, Spigelia, Strontium carb, *Sulphur*.

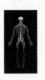

NERVE

Neuralgia

ACONITUM, Actea spicata, *Agaricus*, *Ammonium mur*, ARSENICUM, Berberis, Calc carb, Causticum, CHAMOMILLA, Chelidonium, CIMICIFUGA, COLOCYNTHIS, Dulcamara, Formica rufa, *Gelsemium*, Gnaphalium, Guaiacum, Hecla lava, HYPERICUM, Iris, KALMIA, *Rhododendron*, RHUS TOX, Ruta, Sanguinaria, *Staphysagria*, *Spigelia*, Strontium carb, Sulphur, Tellurium, Viola.

Numbness

Aconitum, Aesculus, Agaricus, Ammonium mur, *Apis*, *Argentum nit*, Arnica, Arsenicum, *Belladonna*, BERBERIS, Bryonia, Calc carb, Calc phos, *Causticum*, *Chamomilla*, *Chelidonium*, *Cimicifuga*, COCCULUS, Colchicum, Colocynthis, Dulcamara, Formica rufa, *Gelsemium*, *Gnaphalium*, *Guaiacum*, *Hypericum*, *Ignatia*, Iris, *Kalmia*, Lachesis, *Ledum*, LYCOPODIUM, *Nat mur*, *Nux vomica*, *Phosphorus*, Phytolacca, PLUMBUM, *Pulsatilla*, Rhododendron, RHUS TOX, Sanguinaria, *Sepia*, *Silicea*, Staphysagria, Strontium carb, Sulphur, Tellurium.

Paralysis

Arsenicum, CAUSTICUM, *Cocculus*, Colocynthis, Dulcamara, Formica rufa, GELSEMIUM, Kalmia, Lachesis, Nux vomica, RHUS TOX.

Tingling, Prickling, Asleep

ACONITUM, Argentum nit, Arnica, Arsenicum, Belladonna, *Gelsemium*, GRAPHITES, *Ignatia*, *Kali carb*, Lachesis, *Ledum*, LYCOPODIUM, *Nat mur*, PHOSPHORUS, PULSATILLA, *Rhododendron*, RHUS TOX, Ruta, *Sepia*, *Silicea*, Staphysagria, *Sulphur*, Thuja.

Trembling

Aconitum, *Agaricus*, *Apis*, *Argentum nit*, Arnica, ARSENICUM, Belladonna, Bryonia, *Calc carb*, Calc fluor, Calc phos, CAUSTICUM, CHELIDONIUM, *Cimicifuga*, COCCULUS, Colchicum, GELSEMIUM, *Hypericum*, *Ignatia*, Kali carb, *Kalmia*, *Lachesis*, Lycopodium, Mag phos, MERC SOL, Nat mur, NITRIC ACID, NUX VOMICA, *Phosphorus*, PLUMBUM, *Pulsatilla*, Ranunculus, Rhododendron, RHUS TOX, Sanguinaria, Sepia, *Silicea*, Spigelia, Staphysagria, Strontium carb, *Sulphur*, Viola.

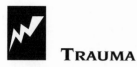
Trauma

Injury, Trauma

Aconitum, Ammonium mur, Apis, Argentum nit, ARNICA, Belladonna, BELLIS, Bryonia, Calc carb ,Calc phos, CALENDULA (skin), Causticum, Chamomilla, Dulcamara, Formica rufa, Hamamelis, Hecla lava, HYPER-ICUM, Kali carb, Kalmia, Lachesis, Ledum, Lycopodium, Nat carb, Nat mur, Nat sulph (head), Nux vomica, Phosphorus, Phytolacca, PULSATIL-LA, Ranunculus, Rhododendron, RHUS TOX, Ruta, Sepia (back), Silicea, Sticta (falls), Spigelia, Staphysagria, Strontium carb, Sulphur, SYMPHY-TUM (bone), Tellurium (spine or sacrum), Thiosinaminum (scarring).

Injury: after-effects or in the remote past

Any of the above trauma remedies, but especially or initially:
ARNICA or HYPERICUM or RHUS TOX in high potency (200, 1M or 10M)
Nat sulph (head injury).

Bruising

ARNICA, BELLIS, Hamamelis, Lachesis, LEDUM, Ruta, Sulphuric acid, Symphytum (bone).

Concussion

Aconitum, ARNICA, Belladonna, Bellis, Bryonia, Calc carb, Calendula, Causticum, Cocculus, Hamamelis, HYPERICUM, Lachesis, Ledum, Lycopodium, Nat mur, NAT SULPH, Nux vomica, Pulsatilla, Rhus tox, Ruta, Sepia, Silicea, Spigelia, Staphysagria, Sulphur, Symphytum.

Cuts

Arnica, Calendula, Hamamelis, Hypericum, Lachesis, Ledum, Phosphorus, Pulsatilla, Silicea, STAPHYSAGRIA, Sulphur, Sulphuric acid.

Dislocation

Aconitum, Agaricus, Ammonium mur, ARNICA, Arsenicum, Belladonna, Bryonia, CALC CARB, Calc fluor, Calc phos, Causticum, Chamomilla, Chelidonium, Cocculus, Colocynthis, Dulcamara, Formica rufa, Kali carb, Lachesis, Ledum, LYCOPODIUM, NAT CARB, NAT MUR, Nux vomica, PHOSPHORUS, PULSATILLA, Ranunculus, Rhododendron, RHUS TOX, Ruta, Sepia, Spigelia, Staphysagria, Strontium carb, Sulphur.

Eye Injury

ACONITUM, Arnica, *Calc carb*, Calendula, *Euphrasia*, Hamamelis, Hypericum, Lachesis, *Ledum*, Nux vomica, *Pulsatilla*, *Rhus tox*, Ruta, STAPHYSAGRIA, Silicea, Sulphur, SYMPHYTUM. (Ruta and Symphytum for the eyeball and socket, Aconitum and Staphysagria for scratches or wounds to the cornea, Ledum for bruising, Silicea for foreign bodies.)

Fracture

ARNICA, followed by LEDUM and SYMPHYTUM.

Bryonia (pain), Calc phos (healing), Sticta (pain), Hypericum (pain or nerve injury), RUTA, *Silicea* (healing).

Also: Bellis, Calc carb, *Calc fluor*, *Calendula*, *Lachesis*, Lycopodium, Phosphorus, Pulsatilla, Rhus tox, *Staphysagria*, *Strontium carb*, Sulphur.

Nerve Injury

Allium cepa, ARNICA, Bellis, Calendula, HYPERICUM, Ledum, Mag phos, *Phosphoric acid*, *Phosphorus*. Hypericum and Arnica in alternation.

Puncture Wounds

APIS, HYPERICUM, Lachesis, LEDUM, Silicea, Sulphur, Symphytum.

Sprains

Aconitum, Agaricus, ARNICA, Arsenicum, Belladonna, *Bellis*, *Bryonia*, CALC CARB, Calc fluor, Calc phos, Calendula, Causticum, *Colocynthis*, Formica rufa, Guaiacum, *Hypericum*, *Ignatia*, Lachesis, *Ledum*, LYCOPODIUM, MILLEFOLIUM, NAT CARB, NAT MUR, NUX VOMICA, PHOSPHORUS, *Pulsatilla*, Radium bromatum, Rhododendron, RHUS TOX, RUTA, Sepia, Silicea, Spigelia, Staphysagria, *Sulphur*, *Symphytum*, Thuja.

Surgery

Aceticum acid, *Aconitum*, Allium cepa, Apis, ARNICA, BELLIS, Berberis, Calc fluor, Calc phos, Calendula, Carbo veg, China, Hamamelis, *Hypericum*, Ledum, Nux vomica, Rhus tox, Ruta, STAPHYSAGRIA, Sticta (insomnia after), *Strontium carb* (shock), Thiosinaminum (scarring).

Wounds

Agaricus, *Apis*, *Argentum nit*, Arnica, Arsenicum, BELLADONNA, Bellis, *Bryonia*, Calc carb, Calc phos, *Calendula*, *Causticum*, *Chamomilla*, DULCAMARA, Hamamelis, HYPERICUM, Kali carb, *Lachesis*, LEDUM, Lycopodium, Millefolium, Nat mur, *Nat sulph*, *Nux vomica*, *Phosphorus*, Phytolacca, *Pulsatilla*, Rhus tox, Ruta, Silicea, *Staphysagria*, Strontium carb, Sulphur.

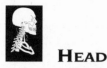

HEAD

Cluster Headache
Belladonna, Nat mur.

Head Injury
Aconitum, ARNICA, Belladonna, Bellis, *Calc carb*, Calc phos (fracture), Cicuta (convulsions), *Hamamelis*, Helleborus, HYPERICUM, Ledum, *Nat mur*, NAT SULPH, Pulsatilla, Rhus tox, *Silicea*, Symphytum (skull fracture).

Menstrual Headache
Belladonna, Cimicifuga, Cocculus, Lachesis, Nat mur, Pulsatilla, Sanguinaria, Sepia.

Migraine
Argentum nit, Arsenicum, Belladonna, Bryonia, CALC CARB, Chamomilla, *Cimicifuga*, COCCULUS, COLOCYNTHIS, *Gelsemium, Guaiacum, Iris, Kali bich*, Kali carb, *Lachesis*, Lycopodium, *Nat mur*, NUX VOMICA, PULSATILLA, SANGUINARIA, SEPIA, Silicea, Spigelia, Sulphur.
Acute: Argentum nit, Belladonna, Gelsemium, Glonoine.
Chronic: Cocculus, Nat mur, Sepia, Lachesis.

Tension / Muscular Contraction Headache
Cimicifuga, Gelsemium, Nux vomica, Ruta.

TMJ Syndrome
AGARICUS, Calc carb, Calc phos, CAUSTICUM, Chamomilla, Cimicifuga, FORMICA RUFA, Ignatia, Mag phos, Phytolacca, Pulsatilla, *Rhododendron*, Rhus tox, Ruta, SILICEA, SPIGELIA, Sulphur.

Trigeminal or Facial Neuralgia
Aconitum, Gelsemium, Rhus tox, Spigelia.

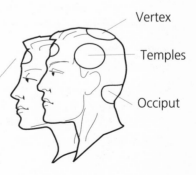

Vertex

Temples

Frontal or Forehead

Occiput

HEADACHE LOCATIONS

Forehead

Aconitum, Aesculus, Agaricus, Ammonium mur, Apis, Argentum nit, ARNICA, Arsenicum, Belladonna, Berberis, Bryonia, Calc carb, Calc phos, Calc carb, Caulophyllum, Causticum, Chamomilla, Chelidonium, Cimicifuga, COCCULUS, Colchicum, Colocynthis, Dioscorea, Dulcamara, Ferrum, Formica rufa, Gelsemium, Guaiacum, IGNATIA, Iris, Kali bich, Kali carb, Kalmia, Lachesis, Ledum, Lycopodium, Nat-mur, Nat sulph, NUX VOMICA, Phosphorus, Phytolacca, PULSATILLA, Ranunculus, Rhododendron, Rhus tox, Ruta, Sanguinaria, Sepia, SILICEA, Spigelia, Staphysagria, Sticta, SULPHUR, Tellurium, Thuja, Viola.

Occiput

Aconitum, Aesculus, Agaricus, Ammonium mur, Apis, Argentum nit, Arnica, Arsenicum, BELLADONNA, Berberis, BRYONIA, Calc carb, Calc phos, CAUSTICUM, Chamomilla, Chelidonium, Cimicifuga, COCCULUS, Colchicum, Colocynthis, Dulcamara, Gnaphalium, Guaiacum, Hypericum, Ignatia, Iris, Lachesis, Lachnantes, Ledum, Lycopodium, Nat mur, Nat sulph, Nux vomica, Phytolacca, Pulsatilla, Ranunculus, Rhododendron, Rhus tox, Ruta, Sanguinaria, Sepia, SILICEA, Spigelia, Staphysagria, Strontium carb, Sulphur, Thuja.

Temples

Aconitum, Agaricus, ARGENTUM, Arnica, Arsenicum, BELLADONNA, BRYONIA, CALC CARB, Causticum, Chamomilla, Chelidonium, COCCULUS, Colchicum, Colocynthis, Dulcamara, Guaiacum, Iris, KALI CARB, Kalmia, Lachesis, Ledum, Lycopodium, NAT MUR, Nux vomica, Phosphorus, Phytolacca, PULSATILLA, Ranunculus, Rhododendron, RHUS TOX, Ruta, SANGUINARIA, Sepia, Silicea, Spigelia, Staphysagria, Strontium carb, Sulphur, THUJA.

Vertex

Aconitum, Actea spicata, Agaricus, APIS, Argentum nit, Arnica, Arsenicum, Belladonna, Bryonia,Calc carb, Calc phos, Causticum, Chamomilla, Chelidonium, Cimicifuga, Cocculus, Colchicum, Colocynthis, Dioscorea, Dulcamara, Ferrum, Formica rufa, Gelsemium, Guaiacum, Hypericum, Ipecac, Iris, Kali carb, Kalmia, Lachesis, Ledum, Lycopodium, Nat carb, Nat mur, Nux vomica, Phosphorus, Phytolacca, Pulsatilla, Ranunculus, Rhododendron, Rhus tox, Ruta, Sanguinaria, Sepia, Silicea, Spigelia, Staphysagria, Sulphur, Tellurium, Thuja.

SPINE

Ankylosing Spondylitis

Initial Stages: AESCULUS, Agaricus, AURUM, Cimicifuga, Conium, Kali carb, KALMIA, Nat mur, PHYTOLACCA, Rhus tox.

Chronic Stages (Ankylosis): Calc carb, CALC FLUOR, Calc phos, CAUS-TICUM, Hecla lava, Silicea (see Arthritic Charts).

Arthritis of the Spine (Spondylosis)

Aconitum, ANT CRUD, Arsenicum, Belladonna, BRYONIA, Calc carb, Calc fluor, Calc phos, Calendula, Carbo veg, Caulophyllum, Causticum, Chamomilla, Chelidonium, CIMICIFUGA, Colchicum, Dulcamara, Ferrum, Gelsemium, Guaiacum, Kali bich, Lachesis, Lycopodium, Nat mur, NUX VOMICA, Phytolacca, Pulsatilla, Ranunculus, RHODODENDRON, RHUS TOX, Ruta, Sanguinaria, Silicea, Sulphur.

Injury / Falls / Blows

Aconitum, Apis, ARNICA, Belladonna (hemorrhage), BELLIS, Bryonia, CALC CARB (lower spine), Calc phos, Cimicifuga, Conium, HYPERICUM, Ignatia, Kali carb, Lycopodium, Nat sulph, Nux vomica (spinal cord), Rhus tox, RUTA, Sepia, SILICEA, Symphytum, Tellurium, Thuja, Zincum.

Lifting Injuries

Arnica, Bellis, Bryonia, CALC CARB, Calc phos, Causticum, Cocculus, Colocynthis, Conium, Dulcamara, Formica rufa, Kali carb, Kalmia, Lachesis, Lycopodium, Nat mur, Nat sulph, Nux vomica, Phosphorus, Rhododendron, RHUS TOX, Ruta, Sanguinaria, Sepia, Silicea, Spigelia, Staphysagria, Sulphur.

Scoliosis (Spinal Curvature)

Aesculus, CALC CARB, CALC FLUOR, CALC PHOS, Causticum, Hecla lava, Lycopodium, Phosphoric acid, Phosphorus, Pulsatilla, Rhus tox, Ruta, Sepia, SILICEA, Staphysagria, SULPHUR, Thuja.

Right Scoliosis: SILICEA, SULPHUR.

Left Scoliosis: CALC PHOS, Thuja.

Spina Bifida

Arnica, Arsenicum, Baryta carb, Belladonna, Bryonia, CALC CARB, CALC PHOS, Dulcamara, Graphites, Hepar sulph, Lachesis, Lycopodium, Phosphorus, PSORINUM, Ruta, SILICEA, Staphysagria, Sulphur.

Spinal Tenderness

AGARICUS, Arsenicum, Belladonna, Berberis, Calc phos, Cimicifuga, COCCULUS, Colocynthis, Hypericum, Lachesis, Nat mur, Ranunculus, Rhus tox, Sepia, SILICEA, Sulphur, Tellurium.

Vertebral Pain

Aconitum, Arnica, Belladonna, CALC CARB, Chelidonium, Cocculus, Dulcamara, Kali carb, Ledum, Lycopodium, Nux vomica, Phosphorus, PULSATILLA, RHUS TOX, Ruta, Sepia, SILICEA, Staphysagria, SULPHUR.

CERVICAL SPINE

General Affinity

Aconitum, Agaricus, BRYONIA, Calc carb, Calc phos, Causticum, CHE-LIDONIUM, Chamomilla, Cimicifuga, Kali carb, Kalmia, Lachnantes, Lycopodium, Nat mur, Pulsatilla, Ranunculus, *Rhododendron*, RHUS TOX, RUTA, SILICEA, SULPHUR.

Cervical Arthritis, Arthrosis

Calc phos, Causticum, Cimicifuga, Lachnantes, Phytolacca, Rhododendron, Ruta.

Cervical or Brachial Neuralgia

Aconitum, Ammonium mur, Arsenicum, Belladonna, Berberis, Bryonia, *Calc carb*, Calc phos, *Chamomilla*, CHELIDONIUM, *Cimicifuga*, Cocculus, COLOCYNTHIS, Ferrum, Formica rufa, Gnaphalium, *Guaiacum*, HYPER-ICUM, KALMIA, *Lachnantes*, *Lycopodium*, Nux vomica, Phosphorus, Pulsatilla, Ranunculus, *Rhododendron*, RHUS TOX, Stellaria, VERATRUM ALBUM.

Cervical Disc Syndrome

Bryonia (all remedies included in Torticollis, Cervical Neuralgia, and Cervical Arthritis may be useful).

Scalenus Anticus Syndrome

Bryonia, INULA HELENIUM (Elecampane), Kreosotum, Mercurius, Plumbum, Sarsaparilla (see remedies under Brachial Neuralgia).

Torticollis

Aconitum, Agaricus, Arnica, Arsenicum, *Belladonna*, Bryonia, *Calc carb*, Calc phos, Caulophyllum, *Causticum*, Chamomilla, Chelidonium, *Cimicifuga*, Cocculus, *Colchicum*, Dulcamara, GUAIACUM, Kalmia, Lachesis, LACHNANTES, LYCOPODIUM, Nat mur, NUX VOMICA, *Phytolacca*, Pulsatilla, Ranunculus, Rhododendron, *Rhus tox*, Ruta, Silicea, Sticta, Sulphur.

Whiplash (Neck Injury)

Arnica, Bryonia, CALC CARB, Calc fluor (chronic), Causticum, Hypericum, Nat sulph, RHUS TOX, Ruta.

THORACIC SPINE

General Affinity
Aesculus, *Agaricus*, Ammonium mur, *Belladonna*, Berberis, *Bryonia*, CALC CARB, *Calc phos*, *Causticum*, Chamomilla, *Chelidonium*, *Cimicifuga*, Cocculus, Colchicum, Colocynthis, Dulcamara, *Guaiacum*, Hypericum, *Kali carb*, *Kalmia*, Lachesis, *Ledum*, *Lycopodium*, Nat mur, Nat sulph, Nux vomica, Phytolacca, PULSATILLA, *Ranunculus*, *Rhododendron*, Rhus tox, Ruta, Sanguinaria, *Sepia*, Silicea, *Spigelia*, Staphysagria, Strontium *carb*, SULPHUR, Tellurium.

Costochondral Subluxations, Chondritis
Agaricus, Bryonia, Causticum, Kalmia, Ranunculus.

Herpes Zoster
Apis, Dulcamara, Iris vers, Kalmia, Mezereum, Nat mur, *Ranunculus*, RHUS TOX.

Intercostal or Post-Herpetic Neuralgia / Pleurodynia
Aconitum, Aesculus, Arnica, Arsenicum, Belladonna, *Bryonia*, Chelidonium, *Cimicifuga*, Kalmia, Mag phos, Mezereum, Nat mur, Nux vomica, Pulsatilla, RANUNCULUS, Rhododendron, R*hus tox*, Spigelia.

Intercostal Rheumatism
Aconitum, Argentum nit, Berberis, Bryonia, Causticum, Cimicifuga, Colchicum, Guaiacum, KALMIA, Lachesis, Lycopodium, N*ux vomica*, *Phosphorus*, Phytolacca, *Pulsatilla*, RANUNCULUS, *Rhododendron*, RHUS TOX, SPIGELIA, Sulphur.

Kyphosis (forward curvature of thoracic spine)
Aconitum, Belladonna, Bryonia, CALC CARB, Causticum, Colocynthis, Dulcamara, Lachesis, Lycopodium, Phosphorus, Pulsatilla, R*hus tox*, R*uta*, Sepia, SILICEA, Staphysagria, SULPHUR, Thuja.

Thoracic Curvature
Aconitum, Belladonna, Bryonia, CALC CARB, Causticum, Colocynthis, Dulcamara, Hepar sulph, Lachesis, Lycopodium, Phosphorus, PULSATILLA, RHUS TOX.

Lumbar Spine

Disc Herniation

Acute: AESCULUS, Agaricus, Arnica, Berberis, BRYONIA, Colocynthis, Cuprum, HYPERICUM, Kali carb, Lachnantes, Rhus tox, Ruta, Tellurium. (See Low Back Pain Charts).

Chronic: Aesculus, CALC FLUOR, Causticum, RHUS TOX, RUTA.

Facet Syndrome

All remedies indicated under low back pain, particularly tissue remedies such as Ruta, Rhus tox, Causticum, and Calc fluor.

Low Back Pain

Actea spicata, Aesculus, Agaricus, Ammonium mur, Arnica, Arsenicum, Belladonna, BERBERIS, Bryonia, CALC CARB, Calc fluor, Caulophyllum, Cimicifuga, Colocynthis, Dulcamara, Formica rufa, Gnaphalium, Guaiacum, Iris vers, KALI CARB, Kalmia, Lachnantes, Lycopodium, Nat mur, Nat sulph, NUX VOMICA, Phytolacca, Pulsatilla, Ranunculus, Rhododendron, RHUS TOX, RUTA, Sepia, Silicea, Staphysagria, Stellaria, Strontium carb, SULPHUR, Tellurium.

Lumbar Curvature

BELLADONNA, Calc carb, CALC PHOS (scoliosis or lordosis), Calc sulph, Phosphorus (lordosis or forward curvature of low back).

Lumbar Neuralgia

AESCULUS, Agaricus, Arsenicum, Berberis, Bryonia, CHAMOMILLA, Cimicifuga, Colocynthis, Guaiacum, KALI CARB, LYCOPODIUM, Nat mur, Nux vomica, Pulsatilla, Rhododendron, RHUS TOX, Silicea, SEPIA, Tellurium.

Lumbosacral Joint

ACONITUM, AESCULUS, Arnica, Arsenicum, Bryonia, Chamomilla, CHELIDONIUM, Colchicum, Gelsemium, Nat sulph, NUX VOMICA, PHOSPHORUS, Silicea.

Sacrum

Actea spicata, AESCULUS, AGARICUS, Arsenicum, Belladonna, BERBERIS, CALC CARB, Calc phos, Chamomilla, Cimicifuga, Colocynthis, Dulcamara, Gelsemium, Guaiacum, Hypericum, Kali carb, Lachnantes, LYCOPODIUM, Nat mur, Nat sulph, Phytolacca, PULSATILLA, Rhus tox, SEPIA, Silicea, TELLURIUM.

Sacroiliac Joint

AESCULUS, Ammonium mur, Argentum nit, Bryonia, CALC PHOS, Cimicifuga, Colocynthis, Gelsemium, Lachnantes, Nux vomica, Phosphorus, Pulsatilla, Rhus tox, Rumex crispus, Sepia, Sulphur, Thuja.

Sciatica

Acute: Aconitum, Agaricus, Arnica, Arsenicum, Belladonna, Berberis, BRYONIA, Chamomilla, Chelidonium, Cimicifuga, COLOCYNTHIS, Dioscorea, Gelsemium, Ginseng, Gnaphalium, HYPERICUM, Iris vers, Kalmia, Lachnantes, MAG PHOS, NUX VOMICA, Plumbum, Pulsatilla, Ranunculus, Rhododendron, Spigelia, Staphysagria, TELLURIUM.

Chronic: Ammonium mur, Argentum nit, Arsenicum, Calc carb, Calc phos, Causticum, Cocculus, Guaiacum, Lachesis, Ledum, Lycopodium, Nat mur, Nat sulph, Phosphorus, Phytolacca, Rhododendron, RHUS TOX, Ruta, Sepia, Silicea, Sulphur, Thuja.

Right Sciatica

Belladonna, Chelidonium, Colocynthis, Dioscorea, Lachesis, Ledum, LYCOPODIUM, Mag phos, Phytolacca, Rhus tox, Sepia, Tellurium.

Left Sciatica

Ammonium mur, Causticum, Chamomilla, Cimicifuga, Colocynthis, Hypericum, Iris vers, Kali bich, Kali carb, Lachesis, Ledum, Nat sulph, Phosphorus, Pulsatilla, Rhus tox, Silicea, Sulphur, Tellurium, Thuja.

Spondylosis, Arthrosis

Calc fluor, Causticum, Cimicifuga, Silicea, Rhus tox.

Coccyx (tailbone) Pain

Aesculus, Agaricus, AMMONIUM MUR, Arnica, Arsenicum, Belladonna, Bellis, Bryonia, CALC CARB, Calc phos, CAUSTICUM, Colocynthis, HYPERICUM, Kali bich, Kali carb, Lachesis, Ledum, Nat sulph, Phosphorus, RHUS TOX, Ruta, Sepia, SILICEA, Sulphur.

SHOULDER

General Affinity, Pain Syndromes

Agaricus, Arsenicum, Bryonia, Calc carb, *Causticum*, CHELIDONIUM, Cimicifuga, FERRUM, Kalmia, Ledum, Lycopodium, Nux vomica, Phytolacca, Pulsatilla, Ranunculus, Rhododendron, RHUS TOX, Staphysagria, SANGUINARIA, SULPHUR.

Right Shoulder

Apis, Berberis, Bryonia, *Calc carb*, CHELIDONIUM, Cimicifuga, *Colocynthis*, FERRUM, *Guaiacum*, Iris vers, *Kali carb*, *Kalmia*, *Ledum*, *Lycopodium*, *Phytolacca*, Pulsatilla, Ranunculus, SANGUINARIA, *Sticta*, Strontium carb.

Left Shoulder

Aconitum, *Aesculus*, *Agaricus*, *Argentum nit*, Chamomilla, Colocynthis, Ferrum, Guaiacum, Kali carb, *Kalmia*, LEDUM, Nat mur, *Rhus tox*, SULPHUR,

Bursitis / Tendonitis

Acute: *Apis*, Arsenicum, *Bellis*, Bryonia, *Chelidonium*, Colocynthis, Ferrum, Ferrum phos, *Kalmia*, Pulsatilla, RUTA, *Sticta*.

Chronic: Phytolacca, Rhododendron, *Rhus tox*, *Ruta*, Sanguinaria, SILICEA, *Sulphur*.

Calcific Deposits, Osteophytes

Calc carb, CALC FLUOR, Hecla lava, Nat mur, *Rhododendron*, *Ruta*, SILICEA.

Contraction of Tendons, Muscles

Agaricus, *Arsenicum*, *Belladonna*, Kali carb, Lycopodium, Mag carb, Nux vomica, Phosphorus, Ranunculus, Rhododendron, Rhus tox.

Frozen Shoulder

Chelidonium, Ferrum Guaiacum, *Phytolacca*, Ruta, *Rhus tox*, Sanguinaria. CALC FLUOR alternating with THIOSINAMINUM.

Rheumatism of Shoulder

Aconitum, Agaricus, Apis, Arsenicum, *Berberis*, Bryonia, Calc carb, *Calc phos*, *Causticum*, *Chelidonium*, Cimicifuga, COLCHICUM, *Colocynthis*, DULCAMARA, FERRUM, Formica rufa, *Guaiacum*, Iris vers, *Kali carb*, Kalmia, Lachesis, *Ledum*, Lycopodium, *Nat mur*, Nux vomica, *Phosphorus*, *Phytolacca*, *Pulsatilla*, *Ranunculus*, RHODODENDRON, RHUS TOX, *Sanguinaria*, SIL-

ICEA, *Staphysagria*, Stellaria, *Sticta*, Strontium carb, SULPHUR, Viola.

Trauma

Arnica, Bryonia, Calc carb, Ferrum, *Rhus tox*, RUTA.

Weakness or Lameness of Shoulder

Aesculus, Bryonia, Causticum, Cimicifuga, *Lachesis*, Lycopodium, Nat mur, Nux vomica, Phytolacca, *Pulsatilla*, Rhododendron, *Rhus tox*, RUTA, Sepia, Staphysagria.

 # ELBOW

Affinity in General / Pain Syndromes

Aconitum, Aesculus, Agaricus, Arsenicum, Bellis, *Bryonia*, Calc carb, Calc phos, Caulophyllum, *Causticum*, Chamomilla, Chelidonium, Cimicifuga, Colchicum, *Colocynthis*, Dulcamara, Ferrum, Formica rufa, Gelsemium, *Guaiacum*, Hypericum, Iris vers, *Kali bich*, Kali carb, KALMIA, Lachesis, Ledum, *Lycopodium*, Nat sulph, Nux vomica, Phytolacca, Pulsatilla, Ranunculus, RHUS TOX, RUTA, Sepia, *Silicea*, Strontium carb, Sulphur, Symphytum, Tellurium, Viola.

Arthritis

Aconitum, Aesculus, Arsenicum, *Bryonia*, Calc carb, Causticum, *Colchicum*, Colocynthis, *Ferrum*, Formica rufa, Guaiacum, Hypericum, Iris vers, *Kali bich*, Kalmia, Lachesis, Ranunculus, Rhus tox, Sepia, Silicea.

Tennis Elbow (Lateral Epicondylitis)

Agaricus, Arnica, Bellis, *Bryonia*, *Calc carb*, Calc phos, CAUSTICUM, Chelidonium, Guaiacum, Hypericum, Kali carb, Kalmia, Rhododendron, RHUS TOX, RUTA, Silicea, Symphytum, Thiosinaminum.

Trauma

Arnica, BRYONIA, *Calc carb*, *Hypericum*, RHUS TOX, RUTA, Silicea, *Strontium carb*.

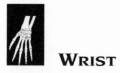

WRIST

Wrist (Affinity in General)

Aconitum, *Actea spicata*, Agaricus, *Argentum nit*, Arsenicum, Belladonna, BELLIS, Bryonia, *Calc carb*, Calc fluor, Calc phos, *Caulophyllum*, CAUS-TICUM, Chamomilla, Chelidonium, Cimicifuga, Cocculus, Colchicum, Colocynthis, Dulcamara, Ferrum, Formica rufa, Gelsemium, GUA-IACUM, *Hypericum*, *Kali bich*, *Kalmia*, Ledum, *Lycopodium*, Nat sulph, *Pulsatilla*, *Rhododendron*, RHUS TOX, RUTA, Silicea, Stellaria, Sticta, SULPHUR, *Viola*.

Right Wrist: Actea spicata, Calc phos, Cimicifuga, Colchicum,*Lycopodium*, *Rhus tox*, Sulphur, VIOLA.

Left Wrist: *Guaiacum*, Ferrum, Kalmia.

Arthritic Nodosities

Ammonium mur, *Calc carb*, *Ledum*, Lycopodium, Rhododendron, *Ruta*.

Arthritis of Wrist

Actea spicata, Aesculus, *Caulophyllum*, Chelidonium, *Colchicum*, Formica rufa, *Guaiacum*, *Kali bich*, Kalmia, *Lachesis*, Pulsatilla, RHUS TOX, RUTA, Sticta, *Viola*.

Carpal Tunnel Syndrome

Actea spicata, Arnica, Bellis, *Calc phos*, *Causticum*, GUAIACUM (left wrist), *Hypericum*, Kalmia, Rhus tox, RUTA, Thiosinaminum, *Viola*.

Ganglion

Ammonium carb, *Benzoic acid*, *Calc carb*, Calc fluor, Rhus tox, RUTA, *Silicea*, Sulphur.

Stiffness of Wrist

Argentum nit, Arsenicum, *Apis*, *Belladonna*, *Chelidonium*, Kali carb, *Ledum*, *Lycopodium*, Nat sulph, *Phosphorus*, Pulsatilla, Rhododendron, RHUS TOX, RUTA, *Sepia*, Staphysagria, *Sulphur*.

Swelling of Wrist

Actea spicata, *Apis*, Bryonia, *Calc carb*, Dulcamara, Kali bich, *Lachesis*, Phosphorus, Rhododendron, RHUS TOX, Sepia, Sticta.

HAND

Hand (Affinity in General)

Actea spicata, Aconitum, Aesculus, Agaricus, Apis, Arsenicum, Belladonna, Benzoic acid, *Calc carb*, Calc phos, Caulophyllum, Chamomilla, Cocculus, *Colchicum*, Gelsemium, *Guaiacum*, *Hypericum*, Kali carb, *Kalmia*, Lachesis, Ledum, Lycopodium, Nat sulph, Nux vomica, Phosphorus, Phytolacca, Pulsatilla, Ranunculus, Rhododendron, RHUS TOX, Ruta, Sanguinaria, Sepia, *Staphysagria*, Stellaria, *Sulphur*, Tellurium, *Viola*.

Arthritis of Hands

Actea spicata, Aesculus, Berberis, CALC CARB, Calc phos, CAULO-PHYLLUM, CAUSTICUM, Chelidonium, COLCHICUM, *Guaiacum*, Lachesis, LEDUM, *Lycopodium*, Phytolacca, *Pulsatilla*, Rhododendron, RHUS TOX, *Ruta*, Sanguinaria, Silicea, *Viola*.

Arthritis of Fingers

Actea spicata, Benzoic acid, Berberis, *Calc carb*, *Caulophyllum*, COLCHICUM, Guaiacum, Hypericum, Kali bich, *Ledum*, Lycopodium, Pulsatilla, *Phytolacca*, *Rhus tox*.

Arthritic Nodosities of Fingers

Aesculus, APIS, BENZOIC ACID, Berberis, CALC CARB, *Calc fluor*, *Calc phos*, *Caulophyllum*, CAUSTICUM, *Colchicum*, Hecla lava, LEDUM, LYCO-PODIUM, *Rhododendron*, Sepia, *Silicea*, Staphysagria, Sulphur, *Urtica urens*.

Dupuytren's Contracture

Actea spicata, Benzoic acid, CALC FLUOR, CAUSTICUM, Gelsemium, *Guaiacum*, Hecla lava, Lycopodium, Nat mur, Ruta, SILICEA, Sulphur, THIOSINAMINUM.

Stiffness of Fingers

Agaricus, Ammonium mur, *Apis*, *Arsenicum*, *Belladonna*, Berberis, Bryonia, *Calc carb*, *Caulophyllum*, *Causticum*, Chamomilla, Cocculus, Colocynthis, Dulcamara, *Ferrum*, Kali carb, LEDUM, LYCOPODIUM, Nat mur, Nat sulph, Nux vomica, Phosphorus, Pulsatilla, RHUS TOX, Sanguinaria, Sepia, *Silicea*, Sulphur.

Writer's Cramp

Aconitum, Agaricus, Argentum nit, *Causticum*, *Cimicifuga*, Gelsemium, Kali carb, MAG PHOS, Ranunculus, Ruta, *Silicea*, Sulphur, Thuja.

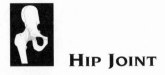

Hip Joint

General Affinity, Pain Syndromes

Aconitum, Actea spicata, Aesculus, Agaricus, Ammonium mur, Apis, Arnica, ARSENICUM, Belladonna, Benzoic acid, Berberis, Bryonia, CALC CARB, Calc fluor, Calc phos, Causticum, Chamomilla, CHELIDONIUM, Cimicifuga, Cocculus, COLCHICUM, COLOCYNTHIS, Ferrum, Formica rufa, Gelsemium, Guaiacum, Hypericum, Kali bich, Kali carb, Kalmia, Lachesis, LEDUM, Lycopodium, Medorrhinum, Nat mur, Nat sulph, Phosphoric acid, Phosphorus, Phytolacca, PULSATILLA, Rhododendron, RHUS TOX, Ruta, Sanguinaria, Sepia, SILICEA, Staphysagria, Sulphur.

Right Hip

Aesculus, Agaricus, Chelidonium, Kali bich, Kali carb, LEDUM, Nat sulph, Phosphorus, Sepia.

Left Hip

Aconitum, Ammonium mur, Apis, Argentum nit, Benzoic acid, CAUSTICUM, Cocculus, Colocynthis, Gelsemium, Iris vers, Lycopodium, Nat sulph, Sanguinaria, Sulphur, THUJA.

Arthritis of Hip

Aconitum, Arnica, Chelidonium, COLCHICUM, Formica rufa, Kali bich, Kalmia, Ledum, Lycopodium, Nat mur, Phosphorus, Phytolacca, Pulsatilla, RHUS TOX, Sanguinaria, Sulphur.

Cramps in the Hip

Belladonna, Causticum, Cimicifuga, Colocynthis, Ledum, Nat mur, Phosphorus, Ruta, Sepia.

Dislocation of Hip

Aesculus, BELLADONNA, BRYONIA, CALC CARB, CALC FLUOR, CAUSTICUM, Colocynthis, Lycopodium, Pulsatilla, Rhus tox, Ruta, Sulphur, Thuja.

Hip Joint disease

Aesculus, AURUM, Bryonia, CALC CARB, Calc phos, Causticum, Colchicum, Colocynthis, Hecla lava, Kali carb, Kalmia, Ledum, Lycopodium, Nat mur, Phosphorus, Phytolacca, PULSATILLA, Rhus tox, Ruta, Sepia, SILICEA, Strontium carb, Sulphur, THUJA.

Injury of Hip

AESCULUS, ARNICA, Bryonia, Calc phos, Rhus tox, Ruta, Silicea.

Stiffness of the Hip

Aconitum, Agaricus, Arsenicum, BELLADONNA, CHAMOMILLA, Colocynthis, Ledum, Lycopodium, Nat mur, Nux vomica, Rhus tox, Sepia, Silicea, Staphysagria, Sulphur.

Tension in Hip

Agaricus, Ammonium mur, Belladonna, Berberis, Bryonia, Calc carb, Cimicifuga, Colocynthis, Lycopodium, Nat mur, Nux vomica, PULSATILLA, Rhus tox, Sepia, Strontium carb, Sulphur, Thuja.

Weakness, Lameness of Hip

AESCULUS, Agaricus, Apis, Bryonia, Calc carb, CALC PHOS, Chamomilla, Cocculus, Kali carb, Rhus tox, RUTA, Sepia, Thuja.

KNEE

Knee (Affinity in General):

Aconitum, Actea spicata, Aesculus, Agaricus, Ammonium mur, APIS, Arnica, Arsenicum, Belladonna, Bellis, BENZOIC ACID (gout), Berberis, Bryonia, CALC CARB, Calc phos, CAUSTICUM, Chamomilla, CHELIDONIUM, Cocculus, Colchicum, Colocynthis, Ferrum, Formica rufa, Gelsemium, Guaiacum, Iris vers, Kali bich, KALI CARB, Kalmia, Lachesis, LEDUM, Lycopodium, Nat mur, Nat sulph, Nux vomica, Phosphorus, PHYTOLACCA, Pulsatilla, Rhododendron, RHUS TOX, Ruta, Sepia, Silicea, Stellaria, Sticta, Strontium carb, Sulphur, Symphytum, Tellurium, Thiosinaminum, Thuja.

Arthritis

Aconitum, Agaricus, Arsenicum, Benzoic acid, Berberis, BRYONIA, CALC CARB, Calc phos, Causticum, Cimicifuga, Cocculus, Dulcamara, Gelsemium, Guaiacum, Hypericum, Kali bich, KALI CARB, Kalmia, Lachesis, Ledum, Lycopodium, Nat mur, Nux vomica, Phosphorus, Phytolacca, Pulsatilla, Ranunculus, Rhododendron, RHUS TOX, Sepia, Sticta, Thuja.

Right Knee: Agaricus, Cimicifuga, Lycopodium, Pulsatilla, Sulphur.

Left Knee: Apis, Benzoic acid, Caulophyllum, Kalmia.

Back of Knee (Popliteal Space)

Arsenicum, BELLADONNA, Bryonia, Causticum, China, Ledum, Lycopodium, Nat carb, NAT MUR, Nux vomica, Phosphorus, Pulsatilla, Rhus tox, Staphysagria, Sulphur, Thuja.

Baker's Cyst

Calc phos, Calc fluor, Ledum, Phosphorus, Pulsatilla, Rhus tox, RUTA, Silicea, Sticta, Sulphur.

Cracking of Knee

Arsenicum, Benzoic acid, Calc carb, CAUSTICUM, Cocculus, Ledum, Nux vomica, Pulsatilla, Sepia, SULPHUR.

Inflammation of Knee (Bursitis, Synovitis, Acute arthritis)

Acute: Aconitum, Arnica, APIS, BRYONIA, Nat mur, Nux vomica, PUL-SATILLA, Sticta.

Chronic: Benzoic acid, Calc carb, Cocculus, Fluoric acid, Guaiacum, Ledum, Lycopodium, Phosphorus, Phytolacca, RHUS TOX, RUTA, Silicea, Sulphur.

Injury of Knee

Apis, Arnica, Bellis, BRYONIA, Calc carb, RHUS TOX, RUTA, Thuja.

Knee Cap (Patella)

BELLADONNA, Bryonia, Calc carb, Causticum, Chelidonium, Ledum, Rhus tox, Spigelia, Staphysagria.

Meniscal Tears

Arnica, CALC FLUOR, Causticum, RUTA (see remedies for Injury)

Osgood-Schlatter

Calc fluor, RUTA (see Arthritis, Inflammation, Swelling in this section).

Shin Splints

Arnica, Bellis, Rhus tox, RUTA, Symphytum (see Trauma, Myalgia, Tendonitis).

Stiffness of Knee

Aesculus, Arsenicum, Belladonna, Berberis, BRYONIA, Calc carb, CAUSTICUM, Chelidonium, Cocculus, Colocynthis, Kali bich, Kali carb, Lachesis, LEDUM, LYCOPODIUM, Nat mur, Nat sulph, Nux vomica, Phosphorus, Phytolacca, Pulsatilla, RHUS TOX, Sanguinaria, Sepia, SILICEA, Spigelia, Staphysagria, SULPHUR.

Swelling at Back of Knee

APIS, Arnica, Belladonna, Benzoic acid, Berberis, Bryonia, Calc carb, Cocculus, Lycopodium, Rhododendron, Silicea.

Swelling of Knee

Aconitum, Aesculus, APIS, Arnica, Arsenicum, Belladonna, Benzoic acid, BERBERIS, BRYONIA, CALC CARB, Calc phos, Causticum, Cocculus, Colchicum, Ferrum, Kali carb, Lachesis, LEDUM, LYCOPODIUM, Nat mur, Nux vomica, Phosphorus, Phytolacca, PULSATILLA, Rhododendron, RHUS TOX, Ruta, Sepia, SILICEA, Sticta, Sulphur.

ANKLE

Ankle (Affinity in General)

Actea spicata, Agaricus, Arnica, Arsenicum, Belladonna, Benzoic acid, Berberis, Bryonia, Calc carb, Calc phos, Caulophyllum, CAUSTICUM, Chamomilla, Chelidonium, Colchicum, Colocynthis, Formica rufa, Gelsemium, Guaiacum, Kalmia, Lachesis, Lachnantes, LEDUM, Lycopodium, Nat mur, Nat sulph, Phosphorus, Phytolacca, Pulsatilla, Ranunculus, Rhododendron, RHUS TOX, RUTA, Sanguinaria, Sepia, Silicea, Spigelia, Stellaria media, Sticta, STRONTIUM CARB, Sulphur, Symphytum, Tellurium, Viola.

Achilles Tendonitis

Aconitum, Aesculus, Agaricus, Arnica, Belladonna, Benzoic acid, Berberis, Bryonia, Calc carb, CAUSTICUM, Chelidonium, Cimicifuga, Colchicum, Colocynthis, Dulcamara, Ignatia, Kali bich, Ledum, Lycopodium, Nat mur, Pulsatilla, Ranunculus, Rhododendron, RHUS TOX, RUTA, Sepia, Staphysagria, SULPHUR, THUJA.

Arthritis of the Ankle

Actea spicata, Calc phos, Caulophyllum, Causticum, Chelidonium, Colchicum, Gnaphalium, Guaiacum, Kalmia, Ledum, Lycopodium, Pulsatilla, Rhododendron, Ruta, Sanguinaria, Silicea, Stellaria, Sticta, Sulphur, Viola.

Restless Leg Syndrome

Calc phos, Causticum, Chamomilla (restless from pain), Lycopodium, Nat mur, Rhus tox, Ruta, Sepia, Staphysagria (restless from pain), Sticta, Sulphur, ZINCUM.

Sprains

ARNICA, Bellis, BRYONIA, Calc carb, Ledum, Nat carb, RHUS TOX, RUTA, Strontium carb, Symphytum.

Weak Ankles

Calc carb, Causticum, Ferrum, NAT CARB, Nat mur, NAT SULPH, RHUS TOX, RUTA, SILICEA, STRONTIUM CARB, Sulphur.

FOOT

Foot Affinity

Actea spicata, Agaricus, Ammonium mur, Apis, Arnica, Arsenicum, Belladonna, Berberis, Calc carb, Caulophyllum, Causticum, Cocculus, Colchicum, Colocynthis, Dulcamara, Gelsemium, Graphites, Guaiacum, Kalmia, Lachesis, Ledum, Lycopodium, Nat mur, Nat sulph, Nux vomica, Phosphorus, Phytolacca, Pulsatilla, Ranunculus, Rhododendron, RHUS TOX, Ruta, Sanguinaria, Sepia, Silicea, Spigelia, Staphysagria, Strontium carb, Sulphur, Thuja.

Arthritis of Foot

Calc carb, Causticum, Colchicum, Guaiacum, Lachesis, LEDUM, Nat sulph, Phosphorus, Phytolacca, Rhododendron, Ruta.

Arthritis of Toes

Actea spicata, AURUM, Benzoic acid, Caulophyllum, Causticum, Colchicum, Gnaphalium, Hypericum, Kali carb, Ledum, Pulsatilla, Silicea, Sticta, Strontium carb.

Back of Foot

Aesculus, Agaricus, Calc carb, CAUSTICUM, Chelidonium, Colocynthis, Ferrum, Guaiacum, Lachesis, Ledum, Nat sulph, Phytolacca, Pulsatilla, Sanguinaria, Silicea.

Bunions: Hypericum, Lycopodium, Rhododendron, SILICEA, Sulphur.

Flat Feet (Fallen Arches)

Calc carb, Calc phos, Guaiacum, Nat carb, Phosphorus, Sepia, Strontium carb, Sulphur.

Heels

Agaricus, Ammonium mur, Arsenicum, Berberis, Calc carb, Calc phos, Caulophyllum, CAUSTICUM, Chamomilla, Chelidonium, Colchicum, Colocynthis, Graphites, Kali carb, LEDUM, Lycopodium, Nat mur, Nat sulph, Phosphorus, Phytolacca, PULSATILLA, Ranunculus, Rhododendron, Rhus tox, Ruta, Sanguinaria, Sepia, Silicea, Sulphur.

Sole

Agaricus, Arsenicum, Berberis, Bryonia, CALC CARB, CAUSTICUM, Cimicifuga, Gelsemium, Guaiacum, Kali carb, LEDUM, Lycopodium, Nat sulph, Phosphorus, PULSATILLA, Ruta, Silicea, SULPHUR, Thuja.

EMOTIONS

Anger, Irritability

Aesculus, Apis, BRYONIA, Caulophyllum, CHAMOMILLA, Chelidonium, Cocculus, COLOCYNTHIS, Gelsemium, Gnaphalium, Kalmia, Lachesis, Nat mur, NUX VOMICA, Ranunculus, Sanguinaria, Strontium carb.

Anxiety or Fear

ACONITUM, Actea spicata, Agaricus, Ammonium mur, Apis, Argentum nit, Arnica, ARSENICUM, BELLADONNA, Berberis, Bryonia, CALC CARB, Calc fluor, Calendula, Caulophyllum, Causticum, Chelidonium, Cimicifuga, Cocculus, Dulcamara, Gelsemium, Hypericum, Iris vers, Kali carb, Kalmia, Lycopodium, Nat mur, Ranunculus, Rhododendron, Rhus tox, RUTA, Sepia, Silicea, Spigelia, Strontium carb, Sulphur, Viola.

Depression

Aesculus, Agaricus, Ammonium mur, Arsenicum, Calc phos, CAUSTICUM, Chelidonium, CIMICIFUGA, Cocculus, Colchicum, Formica rufa, Hypericum, Lachesis, Lachnantes, NAT MUR, NAT SULPH, Phytolacca, Ruta, SEPIA, Spigelia, Strontium carb, Sulphur.

MODALITIES

PHYSICAL MODALITIES

< Motion
Aesculus, Actea spicata, Berberis, BRYONIA, Calc phos, Caulophyllum, Cocculus, COLCHICUM, Colocynthis, Dulcamara, Guaiacum, Kali bich, Kalmia, Ledum, Nat mur, Nux vomica, Phytolacca, Ranunculus, Silicea. Sticta.

Pain on Beginning to Move
Causticum, Lachesis, Ledum, LYCOPODIUM, PHOSPHORUS, PULSATIL-LA, Rhododendron, RHUS TOX, Ruta, Silicea, Thuja.

Pain < First motion > Continued Motion
Agaricus, Causticum, FERRUM, Lachesis, LYCOPODIUM, Medorrhinum, PULSATILLA, Rhododendron, RHUS TOX, Ruta, Thuja.

> Motion
Argentum nit, Bellis, Causticum, Chamomilla, China, Dulcamara, Ferrum, Kali carb, Kali sulph, Lachesis, Lycopodium, Nat sulph, PULSATILLA, RHODODENDRON, RHUS TOX, Ruta, Sepia, Stellaria, Thuja.

TEMPERATURE MODALITIES

> Warmth
Aesculus, Agaricus, ARSENICUM, Bryonia, Calc phos, Causticum, Chamomilla, Colchicum, Colocynthis, Kali carb, Kalmia, Lycopodium, Nux vomica, Phytolacca, Rhododendron, RHUS TOX, SILICEA, Sulphur.

< Warmth of Bed
Apis, LEDUM, Phytolacca, Stellaria, Sulphur

< Warmth
Apis, Bryonia, Guaiacum, Pulsatilla, Sepia, Stellaria, Sulphur.

> Warmth of Bed
ARSENICUM, Lycopodium, Nux vomica, RHUS TOX.

> Cool Bathing
Apis, Guaiacum, LEDUM, PULSATILLA, Stellaria.

< Getting Cold or Chilled
ARSENICUM, Belladonna, Bryonia, Calc carb, Calc phos,Colchicum, Kalmia, NUX VOMICA, Pulsatilla, Ranunculus, RHUS TOX.

WEATHER MODALITIES

< Wet Weather, Damp

Argentum nit, ARSENICUM, Belladonna, Bryonia, CALC CARB, Calc fluor, Calc phos, Causticum, Chamomilla, Cimicifuga, Colchicum, DULCAMA-RA, Ferrum, Formica rufa, Gelsemium, Hamamelis, Hepar sulph, Hypericum, Kali carb, Kalmia, Lachesis, Lycopodium, Nat mur, NAT SULPH, Nux vomica, Phytolacca, PULSATILLA, Ranunculus, RHODODENDRON, RHUS TOX, Ruta, Sanguinaria, Sepia, Silicea, Spigelia, Staphysagria, Sticta, Sulphur, Thuja.

> Wet weather

Aconitum, Arsenicum, Belladonna, BRYONIA, CAUSTICUM, Chamomilla, MEDORRHINUM, NUX VOMICA, Rhododendron, Sepia, Silicea, Spigelia, Staphysagria, Sulphur.

< Change of Weather

Aconitum, Actea spicata, Apis, Arsenicum, Belladonna, Benzoic acid, BRYONIA, Calc carb, Calc fluor, Calc phos, Causticum, Chamomilla, Chelidonium, Cocculus, Colchicum, DULCAMARA, Gelsemium, Hypericum, Kali carb, Kalmia, Lachesis, Nat mur, Nat sulph, Nux vomica, Phytolacca, Pulsatilla, RANUNCULUS, RHODODENDRON, RHUS TOX, Ruta, SILICEA, Sanguinaria, Sepia, Spigelia, Sticta, Strontium carb, Sulphur.

Condition Caused by Getting Wet

Belladonna, Bryonia, CALC CARB, CHAMOMILLA, Dulcamara, Lycopodium, Nux vomica, Pulsatilla, RHUS TOX, Sepia, Silicea, Spigelia, Strontium carb, Staphysagria, SULPHUR.

COMBINED MODALITIES

> Motion > Warmth

Agaricus, Causticum, Chamomilla, Ferrum, Kali carb, Lycopodium, Rhododendron, RHUS TOX, Stellaria.

> Motion < Warmth

Kali sulph, PULSATILLA, Sepia, Thuja.

< Motion > Warmth

Aesculus, BRYONIA, Calc phos, COLCHICUM, Colocynthis, Kali bich, Kalmia, Nux vomica, Phytolacca, SILICEA.

< Motion < Warmth (Bed or Applications)

Bryonia, Guaiacum, Ledum, Phytolacca.

BACK PAIN MODALITIES

POSTURE AND MOTION

Pain from Exertion
Agaricus, Berberis, Bryonia, Calc carb, Calc phos, Causticum, Cocculus, Hypericum, Kali carb, Lycopodium, Ruta, Sepia, Sulphur.

Pain from Lifting
CALC CARB, Calc phos, LYCOPODIUM, Nat mur, *Nux vomica,* RHUS TOX, Ruta, Sanguinaria, *Sepia,* Staphysagria, Sulphur.

< Lying
Agaricus, Arnica, Bellis, *Berberis,* Calc carb, Colocynthis, Dulcamara, Kali carb, Lycopodium, Nat mur, *Nux vomica, Pulsatilla, Rhus tox,* Staphysagria.

< Lying on the Back
Ammonium mur, Apis, Belladonna, Berberis, Bryonia, COLOCYNTHIS, Nat mur, Pulsatilla, Sepia, Staphysagria, Tellurium.

> Lying Down
Agaricus, Arsenicum, Bryonia, Kali carb, *Nat mur, Nux vomica, Ruta,* Sepia, Silicea.

> Lying on the Back
Aesculus, Colchicum, Gnaphalium, *Kali carb,* Lachesis, NAT MUR, Nux vomica, Pulsatilla, *Rhus tox,* RUTA, Sepia, Silicea.

> Lying on Something Hard
Ammonium mur, Belladonna, *Kali carb,* Lycopodium, NAT MUR, Pulsatilla, *Rhus tox, Sepia.*

< Sitting
AGARICUS, Apis, Argentum nit, Belladonna, *Berberis,* Bryonia, *Calc carb,* Calc fluor, *Causticum,* Chamomilla, Cocculus, Dulcamara, *Kali carb,* Lachesis, Ledum, Lycopodium, Nat mur, *Nat sulph,* Nux vomica, Pulsatilla, *Rhododendron,* RHUS TOX, *Ruta,* SEPIA, Silicea, *Sulphur.*

< Rising from Sitting

Aesculus, AGARICUS, Apis, Argentum nit, Arsenicum, BERBERIS, Bryonia, Calc carb, CAUSTICUM, Iris vers, Lachesis, Ledum, Lycopodium, PHOSPHORUS, PULSATILLA, Rhododendron, RHUS TOX, Ruta, Sepia, Silicea, Staphysagria, SULPHUR, Thuja.

Rising from Long Sitting Almost Impossible

Aesculus, Agaricus, Ammonium carb, Belladonna, Berberis, Calc carb, Pulsatilla, RHUS TOX.

< Standing

Aesculus, Agaricus, Belladonna, Berberis, Bryonia, Calc carb, Cocculus, Kali carb, Lycopodium, Nat mur, Nux vomica, Pulsatilla, Ruta, Sepia, SULPHUR.

Can't Stand Erect

Bryonia, Arnica, Belladonna, Nat mur, Rhus tox, SULPHUR, THUJA.

< Stooping

Aesculus, AGARICUS, Berberis, Bryonia, Chamomilla, Chelidonium, Cocculus, Dulcamara, Guaiacum, Kali carb, Lycopodium, Nat mur, Nux vomica, Pulsatilla, Rhododendron, Rhus tox, Ruta, SEPIA, Silicea, Strontium carb, Sulphur.

< Straightening up the Back

Agaricus, Calc carb, Chelidonium, Kali carb, Lachesis, Nat mur, Nux vomica, Sepia, Sulphur.

< Walking

AESCULUS, Agaricus, Ammonium mur, Argentum nit, Belladonna, Bryonia, Causticum, Chamomilla, Chelidonium, Cocculus, Colchicum, Colocynthis, Hypericum, Iris vers, KALI CARB, Lycopodium, Nat mur, Nux vomica, Phytolacca, RANUNCULUS, Rhus tox, Ruta, Sepia, Spigelia, Strontium carb, Sulphur.

> Walking

Argentum nit, Belladonna, Bryonia, Calc fluor, DULCAMARA, Nat mur, Nux vomica, Pulsatilla, RHUS TOX, Ruta, Sepia, Staphysagria, Strontium carb, Tellurium.

TEMPERATURE MODALITIES

> Warm Applications

Calc fluor, Causticum, N*ux vomica*, RHUS TOX.

< Warm Applications

Guaiacum, Pulsatilla, Sulphur.

< Damp Weather

CALC CARB, Calc phos, DULCAMARA, *Phytolacca*, *Rhododendron*, RHUS TOX, Sepia.

Appendix

Remedy Relationships

REMEDY RELATIONSHIPS

There is an inherent relationship between natural substances, some being compatible with each other, while others being entirely antagonistic. This is seen in chemistry, in the plant world, and in the behavior of all insect and animal species. These relationships are seen in a new light in homeopathy, where a subtle interaction between apparently unrelated species, minerals, herbs, and other substances is clearly demonstrated.

The knowledge of these relationships is based on the clinical practice and experience of homeopaths over two centuries with millions of prescriptions. This section tabulates the known relationships between remedies, showing which ones are complementary, antidotal, or incompatible.

Complementary Remedies

Complementary remedies follow each other well, and often help complete the action started by the other. In some cases, a complementary remedy is considered to be deeper than its related remedy. Silicea is the "chronic" of Pulsatilla, and Calc carb is the "chronic" of Belladonna. Where one of these latter remedies works acutely or locally, the complementary chronic remedy may work deeper to change the constitutional tendency. On the other hand, some complements work locally, as a drainage or detoxication factor, to help the action of a deeper, constitutional homeopathic remedy.

Antidotes

Antidotal remedies can partially or wholly interfere with or halt the action of another remedy. This happens if they are used in close proximity to each other or sequentially. Sometimes antidotes are used intentionally to stop the action of a remedy that seems inappropriate. This is best left to a professional homeopath, as it can create confusion in the symptom picture of the individual.

Incompatibles

Some remedies should *never* be used in relation with each other, neither simultaneously or following one another. If they are it can upset the vital force and subtle healing mechanisms of the body. On the other hand, some remedies act as a bridge between incompatibles. One well know relationship is the use of Hepar sulph between the remedies Silicea and Mercurius, which are strongly incompatible.

The following charts outline the relationship of the 61 remedies detailed in this book compared with *all* other homeopathic remedies. For the sake of brevity, the standard abbreviations for these remedies are used. For those totally unfamiliar with these short forms, they can be found in any of the standard materia medica listed in the Resources section at the end of the book. Note that some of the remedies featured in this book are not listed here, since their remedy relationships are not yet well known. These include Actea spicata, Bellis, Stellaria, etc.

There are a few antidotes that bear particular pointing out.

Coffee (coff.) can potentially antidote all homeopathic remedies, but there are a number that are very specifically impacted by drinking coffee or using other forms of caffeine. Such remedies include Belladonna, Causticum, Lycopodium, Nux vomica, Chelidonium, Gelsemium, etc.

Vinegar (acet-ac.) can antidote many remedies including Arnica, Causticum, Colchicum, Colocynthis, Pulsatilla, Ranunculus, Sepia, etc.

Camphor (camph.) antidotes many remedies, particularly Dulcamara, Ledum, Kali carb, Nat mur, Silicea, Staphysagria, Viola, etc.

Chamomile tea (cham.) should not be used with remedies such as Colocynthis, Hypericum, Lachesis, Nux vomica, and Sulphur.

Wine (vitis) is also not advisable when taking remedies which include Arnica, Agaricus and Belladonna.

There are also antagonistic relationships between otherwise effective remedies. For example, Rhus tox and Apis should not be used close to each other, and Bryonia and Pulsatilla don't do well together. It is useful before using any remedy in the materia medica to check its compatibility in the accompanying charts.

DURATION OF REMEDIES
In the charts, the potential duration in days of a number of remedies is listed. This is merely a *comparative* guide to the depth of action of remedies, and is in no way a definite or rigid classification. The actual duration of the a remedy's action is highly variable, depending on the nature of the illness and the person. Also, we continue to learn more about our remedies. Some that were once used largely for acute, short-term conditions (like Aconitum), are now felt to be profound, long-acting medicines. Nevertheless, the durations shown here provide some comparative basis for judging the characteristic depth of the remedy.

Remedy	Antidotes (Incompatibles)	Complementary
Aconitum	camph,. chin., ign., ipec.	arn., bell., berb., bry., **coff.**, mill., phos., spong., **sulph.** 2 days
Aesculus	nux-v.	carb-v., lach., mur-ac.
Agaricus	absin., atro., calc., camph., coff., nit-ac., **puls.**, rhus-t., vitis.	calc. 40 days
Ammonium mur	camph., caust., *coff.*, hep., nux-v.	30 days
Apis	all-c., ars., canth., carb-ac., carb-v., chin., dig., iod., ip., lac-ac., lach., led., nat-m., phos., plan., urt-u. (phos., rhus-t.)	arn., ars., bar-c., hell., merc-cy., **nat-m.**, puls., sars., sulph.
Argentum nitricum	am-caust., ars., bell., calc., cina, iod., lyc., merc., nat-c., **nat-m.,** nux-v., phos., puls., rhus-t., sep., sil., sulph., tab. (coff., vesp.)	calc., nat mur., puls., sep. 30 days
Arnica	acon., am-c., **am-m.,** ars., bell., berb., *camph.*, chin., cic., coff., ferr., ign., *ip.*, nux-v., paris., seneg. sulph. (ac acet., vitus.)	alum., acon., bry., calc., hyper., ip., nat-s., nux-v., psor., rhus-t., sul-ac., sulph., verat. 7 days
Arsenicum album	bry., camph., carb-ac., **carb-v.,** cham., **chin.,** chin-s., dig., euph., **ferr.,** graph., **hep.,** iod., **ip.,** kali-bi., lach., merc., nat-c., nux-m., **nux-v.,** ol-j., op., **phos.,** plb., rhus-t., samb., sulph., tab., **verat.**	all-s., anthr., carb-v., chin., kali-bi., lach., nat-s., **phos.,** puls., pyrog., rhus-t., sec., sulph., thuj. 30 days in chronic cases
Belladonna	acon., arum-t., atro., camph., chin., **coff.,** con., cupr., ferr., gall-ac., **hep.,** *hyos.*, merc., nux-v., **op.,** piloc., plat., plb., puls., sabad., stram., thea., vitis.	bor., calc., hep., merc., nat-m., vario. 1-7 days
Berberis vulgaris	acon., bell., camph.	lyc., mag-m., sulph.

REMEDY	ANTIDOTES (INCOMPATIBLES)	COMPLEMENTARY
Bryonia	*acon.*, **alum.**, ant-t., ac. mur., **calc.**, *camph.*, **cham.**, chel., chin., chlor., clem. *coff.*, ferr., ferr-m., frag., **ign.**, **nux-v.**, **puls.**, *rhus-t.*, seneg. (calc.)	abrot., alum., lyc., nat-m., rhus-t., sep., sulph., upa.

7-21 days |
| Calc carb | bism., **bry.**, camph., chin., chin-s., dig., hep., iod., ip., mez., **nit-ac.**, **nit-s-d.**, **nux-v.**, phos., sep., sulph (bar-c., bry., nit-ac., sulph.) | bell., hep., lyc., rhus-t., sil.

60 days |
Calc fluor		bry., calc., calc. p., kali-mur., nat-mur., **sil.**
Calc phos	(bar-c.)	carb-an., chin., hep., nat-m., ruta, sul-i., sulph., zinc.
Caulophyllum	**(coff.)**	
Causticum	ant-t., **asaf.**, cham., chin., coff., coloc., dulc., euphr., grat., guai., kali-n., *nit-s-d.*, **nux-v.**, pip-m., plb. (acet-ac., cocc., **coff.**, **phos.**)	carb-v., coloc., graph., lach., merc-c., petros., sep., stann., staph.

50 days |
| Chamomilla | *acon.*, all-c., alum., bor., camph., caust., chin., **cocc.**, *coff.*, coloc., com., con., **ign.**, *nux-v.*, **op.**, **puls.**, valer. (nux-v., zinc.) | bell., calc., mag-c., puls., sanic.

20 days |
Chelidonium	acon., all-c., **bry.**, **camph.**, cham., coc-c., coff. **(coff.)**	ars., bry., lyc., merc-d., sulph. 7-14 days
Cimicifuga	**acon.**, bapt., camph., caul., gels., puls.	8-12 days
Cocculus	alco., *camph.*, caps., **cham.**, cupr., ign., merc., *nux-v.*, staph., tab. (caust., **coff.**)	30 days
Colchicum	**bell.**, camph., cocc., led., *nux-v.*, **puls.**, spig., sulph., tab., thuj. (acet-ac.)	ars., carb-v., merc., nux-v., puls., rhus-t., sep., spig.
Colocynthis	*camph.*, caust., cham., cocc., **coff.**, op., *staph.*	caust., kali-c., merc., staph.

7 days |

REMEDY	ANTIDOTES (INCOMPATIBLES)	COMPLEMENTARY
Dulcamara	*camph.*, caps., cupr., ip., kali-c., merc. (acet-ac., bell., lach.)	alum., bar-c., calc., kali-c., nat-s., sulph. 30 days
Gelsemium	atro., bell., chin., coff., dig., nat-m., nux-m., nux-v., puls. (op.)	arg-n., sep. 14 days
Guaiacum	caust., kreos., nux-v., rhus-t., sulph.	40 days
Hypericum	ars., cham., sulph.	7 days
Iris vers	merc., nux-v., phyt.	
Kali carb	**camph.**, coff., dulc., *nit-s-d.*	ars., carb-v., nat-m., nit-ac., nux-v., phos. 50 days
Kalmia	acon., bell., spig.	3 days
Lachesis	alum., am-c., **ars.**, *bell.*, calc., caps., carb-v., cedr., cham., cocc., coff., hep., led., *merc.*, nat-m., nit-ac., nux-v., op., ph-ac., rhus-t., samb., sep., tarent. (acet-ac., **am-c.**, carb-ac., dulc., nit-ac., psor.)	ars., calc., carb-v., crot-c., crot-h., hep., iod., kali-i., lyc., nit-ac., phos. 40 days
Ledum	apis, **camph.**, coff., ip., op., rhus-t. (**chin.**)	sep. 30 days
Lycopodium	**acon.**, camph., caust., cham., chin., **coff.**, graph., lach., nux-v., *puls.* (coff., nux-m., zinc.)	calc., carb-v., chel., graph., ign., iod., ip., kali-c., kali-i., lach., med., nat-m., phos., puls., rhus-t., sulph. 50 d
Nat mur	arg-n., ars., **camph.**, nit-s-d., nux-v., **phos.**, sep.	apis, arg-n., bry., caps., ign., kali-c., lyc., sep., tub. 50 d
Nat sulph	dulc., nit-s-d.	ars. 30 -40 days
Nux vomica	**acon.**, ambr., ars., bell., camph., cham., cocc., **coff.**, dig., euph., *ign.*, iris, lach., op., pall., plat., puls., stram., thuj. (acet-ac., caust., ign., nux-m., tab., zinc.)	bry., cham., con., kali-c., phos., puls., sep., sulph. 7 days

REMEDY	ANTIDOTES (INCOMPATIBLES)	COMPLEMENTARY
Phytolacca	bell., coff., dig., **ign.**, iris, merc., mez., nit-ac., nit-s-d., op., sulph.	sil. 40 days
Pulsatilla	**acet-ac.**, ant-c., ant-t., asaf., bell., calc-p., cench., **cham.**, chin., *coff.*, colch., ign., lyc., nux-v., plat., sabad., stann., stram., sul-ac., sulph. (nux-m)	all-c., arg-n., ars., bry., cham., coff., graph., kali-bi., kali-m., kali-s., lyc., nux-v., sep., sil., stann., sul-ac., sulph., tub., zinc. 40 days
Ranunculus	anac., **bry.**, *camph.*, cham., clem., crot-t., puls., rhus-t. (**acet-ac.**, kali-n., nit-s-d., *staph.*, sulph.)	3 days
Rhododen.	**bry.**, camph., *clem.*, nux-m., nux-v., *rhus-t.*	40 days
Rhus tox	acon., am-c., anac., ant-t., ars., **bell.**, *bry.*, camph., clem., coff., crot-t., cupr., cypr., graph., grin., guai., kali-s., lach., led., merc., mez., plat., plb., ran-b., rhod., sang., sass., sep., sulph., tanac. (apis, **phos.**)	bell., bry., calc., calc-f., caust., lyc., mag-c., med., phos., phyt., puls., sulph., tub. 7 days
Ruta	**camph.**, merc.	calc-p., sil. 30 days
Sanguinaria	op.	ant-t., phos., sars.
Sepia	acet-ac., **acon.**, ant-c., ant-t., calc., chin., merc., merc-c., nat-m., nat-p., *nit-s-d.*, phos., rhus-t., sars., sulph.	gels., ign., kali-c., nat-c., nat-m., nux-v., phos., psor., puls., sabad., sulph. 50 days
Silicea	calc-s., **camph.**, fl-ac., **hep.**, merc., sulph.	calc., caust., fl-ac., hep., lyc., phos., puls., sanic., thuj. 60 days
Spigelia	aur., **camph.**, cocc., merc., *puls.*	spong.
Staphysagria	ambr., **camph.**, merc., thuj. (**ran-b.**)	caust., coloc. 20-30 days
Sticta pulm.	ipec.	

REMEDY	ANTIDOTES (INCOMPATIBLES)	COMPLEMENTARY
Stront. carb	camph.	
Sulphur	acon., ars., camph., caust., cham., *chin*., coff., con., crot-t., hyper., iod., *merc*., nit-ac., nux-v., PULS., rhus-t., *sep*., sil., thuj. (nux-m., ran-b.)	acon., aloe, ars., bad., bell., calc., caust., merc., nux-v., psor., puls., pyrog., rhus-t., sep., sul-i. 40-60 days
Tellurium	nux-v.	
Viola odorata	camph.	

RESOURCES

For a comprehensive list of resources, consult "The Consumer's Guide to Homeopathy" listed in the Introductory Reading section.

HOMEOPATHIC ORGANIZATIONS

National Center For Homeopathy
801 N. Fairfax St. # 306
Alexandria, VA 22314
(703) 548-7790

HOMEOPATHIC PRACTITIONERS

Qualified homeopaths can be found through the following organizations:

National Center For Homeopathy
801 N. Fairfax St. #306
Alexandria, VA. 22314
(703) 548-7790

American Institute of Homeopathy
1585 Glencoe Street #44
Denver CO. 80220
(303) 321-4105

Homeopathic Academy of
Naturopathic Physicians
14653 South Graves Road,
Mulino, OR. 97042
(503) 795-0579

International Foundation
for Homeopathy
2366 Eastlake Ave. #325
Seattle WA. 98102
(206) 324-8230

BOOKS AND TAPES

Many introductory books are available in bookstores, health food stores, etc. Extensive catalogs and descriptions of introductory and advanced books can be obtained from both the mail-order companies listed below.

Homeopathic Educational Services
2036 Blake St.
Berkeley, CA 94704
(800) 359-9051

Minimum Price Books
250 H Street, PO Box 2187
Blaine, WA 98231
(800) 663-8272

INTRODUCTORY READING

Complete Guide to Homeopathy, A. Lockie & N. Geddes, Dorling Kindersley, New York, 1995.

Consumer's Guide to Homeopathy, Dana Ullman, Tarcher, New York, 1995.

Everybody's Guide to Homeopathic Medicines, S. Cummings & D. Ullman, North Atlantic Books, Los Angeles, Tarcher, 1991.

Portraits of Homeopathic Medicines (Volume 1 & 2), C. Coulter, North Atlantic Books, 1986-88.

The Science of Homeopathy, G. Vithoulkas, Grove Press, New York, 1980.

EDUCATIONAL RESOURCES

The following organizations and institutions provide various types of educational programs for laymen and professionals.

Atlantic Academy for Homeopathy
209 First Avenue #2,
New York, NY. 10003
(718) 518-4593

Bastyr University
14500 Juanita Dr.,
Bothell, WA. 98011
(206) 823-1300

British Institute of Homeopathy
(Correspondence Course)
520 Washington Blvd #423
Marina del Rey, CA. 90292
(310) 306-5408

Curentur University
5519 Centinella Ave.
Los Angeles, CA. 90066
(310) 448-1700

Hahnemann Medical Clinic
828 San Pablo
Albany, CA. 94706
(510) 524-3117

Homeopathic Master
Clinician Course
RR #1, F-31
Bowen Island, B.C. VON 1G0
(604) 947-0757

International Foundation for
Homeopathy
PO Box 7
Edmonds, WA. 98020
(206) 776-4147

National College of Naturopathic
Medicine
049 Porter St.
Portland, OR. 97201

Northwestern Academy
of Homeopathy
10700 Old County Road, #15
Minneapolis, MN. 55441
(612) 593-9458

New England School
of Homeopathy
356 Middle Street
Amherst, MA. 01002
(800) 637-4440

The School of Homeopathy
(Correspondence Course)
111 Bala Avenue
Bala Cynwyd, PA. 19004
(610) 667-2927

BIBLIOGRAPHY

Each remedy discussed in this book was compiled with careful reference to over 140 homeopathic materia medica. The following are representative of the texts used in researching this book.

PRINCIPLES

Principles and Practice of Homeopathy, M. Dhawle, D.K. Homeopathic Corporation, Bombay, 1967.
Principles and Art of Cure by Homeopathy, H. A. Roberts, B. Jain, Delhi (Reprint).
Introduction to Homeopathic Prescribing, S. M. Gunavante, B. Jain, Delhi, 1992.
Principles of Prescribing, K. N. Mathur, B. Jain Publishers, Delhi, 1975.

MUSCULOSKELETAL TEXTS

Headache and Its Materia Medica, B. Underwood, Brooklyn, 1888 (Reprint).
Homeopathic Therapeutics of Traumatic Diseases, D. Lakshminarayanan, Shilpa Endowment Trust, Hyderabad, 1988.
Homeopathic Therapy in Gout, Arthritis and Rheumatism, P.S. Kamthan, B. Jain Publishers, New Delhi, 1974.
Musculoskeletal Conditions (12 audio tapes), Robin Murphy, Hahnemann Academy of North America, Pagosa Springs, 1992.
Rheumatic Diseases, S. L. Kumar, B.Jain Publishers, New Delhi, 1986.
Sports Injuries & Exercise Remedies, Steven Subotnik, North Atlantic Books, Berkeley, 1991.
The Rheumatic Remedies, H.A. Roberts, B.Jain, New Delhi, 1939 (Reprint).

GENERAL MATERIA MEDICA

A Study on Materia Medica and Repertory, N. M. Chouduri, B. Jain Publishing, New Delhi, 1929 (Reprint 1991).
Characteristic Materia Medica, Burt, B. Jain, Calcutta, 1873 (Reprint).
Concordant Materia Medica, F. Vermuelen, Merlijn Publishers, Haarlem, 1994.
Characteristic Materia Medica, D. C. Das Gupta, Economic Homeo Pharmacy, Calcutta, 1984.
Characteristics of the Homeopathic Materia Medica, H. Barthal, Barthal & Barthal, Germany, 1987.
Clinical Materia Medica, E. Farrington, Philadelphia, 1887.(Reprint)
Encyclopedia of the Pure Materia Medica (12 Volumes), T. F. Allen, New York, 1874-1879.
Fisches Materia Medicale, Zizu and Guillaume, Editions Boiron, Lyon, 1989.

Guiding Symptoms of Our Materia Medica (10 Volumes), Constantine Hering, Philadelphia, 1879-1891.
Homeopathie Matière Medicale Thérapeutique, Paul Kollistch, Editions Helios, Geneva, 1989.
Materia Medica of New Homeopathic Remedies, O. Julian, Beaconsfield, 1979.
Materia Medica of Homeopathic Medicines, S. R. Phatak, Indian Books and Periodicals, Bombay, 1977.
Materia Medica with Repertory, Wm Boericke, Boericke & Tafel, Santa Rosa, 1927.
Materia Medica Viva, Volume 1-3, G. Vithoulkas, Health and Habitat, Mill Valley, 1992-96.
Physiological Materia Medica, Wm Burt, Chicago, 1883 (Reprint).
Synoptic Materia Medica (Volume 1 & 2), Frans Vermuelen, Merlijn Publishers, Haarlem, 1993.
Synoptic Key of the Materia Medica, C.M. Boger, B. Jain, Calcutta (Reprint).
Studies of Homeopathic Remedies, D.M. Gibson, Beaconsfield Publishers, Beaconsfield, 1987.
The Complete Materia Medica, H Retzek/R. van Zandvoort, Netherlands, 1996.

COMPUTER PROGRAMS

MacRepertory and *ReferenceWorks*, Kent Homeopathic, Fairfax, CA, 1994-96. (Searchable databases of many of the texts listed above).

THERAPEUTIC GUIDES

Homeopathic Emergency Guide, Thomas Kruzel,N.D., North Atlantic Books, Berkeley, 1992.
Homeopathic Therapeutics, W. A. Dewey, 1934 (Reprint).
Pointers to the Common Remedies, M. L. Tyler, (Reprint B. Jain, New Delhi 1990), pp 123-29.
Select Your Remedy, Bishambar Das, New Delhi, 1989.
Textbook of Homeopathic Theory and Practice, George Royal, Jain Publishing, New Delhi, 1982. pp 163-69, 651-56.
Thérapeutique et Repertoire Homeopathiques du Practicien, H. Voison, Librairie Maloine, Paris. 1978.

REPERTORY

Complete Repertory, R. van Zandvoort, Kent Homeopathic, Fairfax, 1994.
Homeopathic Medical Repertory, Robin Murphy N.D.,Hahnemann Academy of North America, Pagosa Springs, 1993.
Boenninghausen's Characteristic Materia Medica and Repertory, C.M. Boger, 1905 (Reprint, B. Jain Publishers, New Delhi, 1993).

GENERAL INDEX

T

Teeth, 124, 171, 191, 198, 234, 247
Teething, 169
Temples, 123, 125, 155, 133, 142, 148, 155, 194, 200, 230, 228, 234, 266
Tenderness, 78, 80, 85, 89, 91, 92, 105, 136, 145, 175, 176, 178, 191, 192, 204, 218, 248, 261, 268
Tendonitis, 76, 102, 103, 110, 155, 161, 167, 171, 172, 173, 189, 205, 215, 217, 221, 224, 226, 227, 229, 258, 260, 273, 281
Tendons, 76, 77, 80, 83, 84, 87, 102, 104, 105, 108, 109, 110, 111, 112, 113, 116, 118, 121, 138, 150, 156, 157, 158, 159, 160, 162, 166, 176, 178, 188, 204, 206, 210, 212, 213, 214, 220, 223, 225, 226, 227, 233, 224, 246, 248, 250, 258, 259, 273
Tennis Elbow, 157, 161, 199, 217, 223, 224, 226, 246, 247, 250, 274
Tenosynovitis, 76, 260
Tension, 76, 78, 81, 88, 90, 92, 93, 94, 95, 102, 103, 105, 106, 107, 109, 111, 122, 123, 138, 139, 143, 152, 154, 155, 156, 166, 168, 170, 172, 173, 180, 185, 188, 195, 206, 212, 213, 222, 223, 235, 236, 243, 244, 252, 261, 265, 278
Thighs, 96, 97, 99, 100, 106, 132, 138, 146, 152, 160, 167, 168, 172, 178, 180, 186, 188, 190, 196, 210, 214, 222, 230, 238, 244, 248
Thoracic, 75, 88, 89, 93, 94, 137, 138,154, 156, 160, 170, 171, 172, 179, 188, 193, 198, 199, 209, 210, 212, 216, 218, 219, 222, 224, 226, 237, 244, 248, 249, 270

Tic Doloreux, 185
Tinnitus, 142, 174, 194, 221, 250
TMJ, 167, 183, 215, 221, 224, 233, 253, 265
Toes, 84, 100, 119, 138, 146, 164, 176, 186, 187, 190, 193, 203, 204, 206, 214, 220, 223, 227, 282
Torticollis, 91, 92, 155, 157, 161, 165, 166, 167, 171, 172, 179, 181, 189, 202, 203, 206, 207, 212, 213, 215, 221, 224, 226, 232, 233, 241, 244, 245, 269
Trauma, 75, 76, 77, 80, 82, 83, 84, 85, 86, 90, 95, 106, 108, 110, 131, 144, 145, 150, 151, 155, 157, 162, 163, 192, 193, 209, 210, 213, 223, 227, 230, 237, 243, 246, 247, 249, 263, 267, 274
Trembling, 80, 81, 105, 109, 118, 121, 123, 124, 125, 130, 132, 136, 137, 140, 142, 143, 146, 158, 160, 164, 165, 166, 172, 174, 184, 192, 193, 195, 198, 204, 209, 216, 223, 244, 252, 262
Tremors, 81, 136, 137, 143, 167
Trigeminal, 179, 234, 235, 265
Trigger, 76, 196
Tumors, 87, 116, 150, 158, 159, 183, 187, 190, 191, 215, 250, 257
Twitching, 80, 81, 94, 100, 105, 121, 130, 136, 137, 146, 166, 172, 180, 185, 192, 196, 206, 209, 212, 223, 230, 234, 242

U

Ulcer, 143, 247
Ulnar, 193, 199, 224
Urethritis, 199
Uric acid, 176, 182, 205, 207 (see Gout)

Uterine, 135, 151, 159, 165, 172,
173, 200, 201, 230, 231, 251

V

Vaccination, 232

Varicose, 87, 134, 135, 151, 159,
163, 191, 217, 231

Veins, 85, 87, 134, 135, 151, 159,
191, 217, 228, 231, 239

Vertebrae, 77, 88, 93, 95, 97, 136,
156, 172, 178, 198, 206, 208, 240,
244

Vertex, 124, 130, 133, 142, 156, 172,
193, 200, 202, 208, 232, 234, 266

Vertigo, 121, 124, 133, 137, 142,
143, 148, 155, 174, 175, 184, 187,
191, 193, 194, 200, 202, 212, 221,
232, 235, 250

W

Weak ankles, 110, 111, 157, 166,
226, 233, 281

Weak joints, 84, 161, 204, 225, 226,
227, 260

Whiplash, 90, 269

Women, 102, 112, 118, 122, 132,
133, 163, 165, 201, 217, 229, 231,
253

Wounds, 83, 85, 162, 237 (see Cuts)

Wrist, 75, 80, 83, 101, 103, 104, 105,
116, 118, 119, 130, 132, 133, 136,
150, 156, 157, 158, 159, 160, 164,
170, 176, 180, 182, 188, 198, 204,
211, 216, 217, 220, 221, 223, 224,
225, 226, 233, 238, 240, 241, 242,
243, 244, 245, 252, 253, 275

REMEDY INDEX

Note: The pages references above refer to the places where information about the remedy can be found in the Materia Medica and Condition Chart sections. To avoid an excessively complex index, it does not include listings from the Therapeutic Guide section.